A Guide to the Formulation of Plans and Goals in Occupational Therapy

This practical guide for occupational therapists introduces a tried and tested method for moving from assessment to intervention, by formulating plans and measurable goals using the influential Model of Human Occupation (MOHO).

Section 1 introduces the concept of formulation – where it comes from, what it involves, why it is important, and how assessment information can be guided by theoretical frameworks and organised into a flowing narrative. Section 2 provides specific instructions for constructing occupational formulations using the Model of Human Occupation. In addition, a radically new way of creating aspirational goals is introduced – based on a simple acronym – which will enable occupational therapists to measure sustained changes rather than single actions. Section 3 presents 20 example occupational formulations and goals, from a wide range of mental health, physical health and learning disability settings, as well as a prison service, and services for homeless people and asylum seekers.

Designed for practising occupational therapists and Occupational Therapy students, this is an essential introduction for all those who are looking for an effective way to formulate plans and goals based on the Model of Human Occupation.

Sue Parkinson practised as an occupational therapist for many years. Sue is the lead author of the Model of Human Occupation Screening Tool (MOHOST) and author of an occupational intervention programme called Recovery through Activity. She works as a freelance trainer providing an online advisory and supervision service.

Rob Brooks is the Course Director for Occupational Therapy at Leeds Beckett University. His clinical practice, teaching, and research have focused on enabling occupational participation for children, young people, and their families.

A Guide to the Formulation of Plans and Goals in Occupational Therapy

Sue Parkinson and Rob Brooks

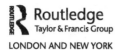
Routledge
Taylor & Francis Group

LONDON AND NEW YORK

First published 2021
by Routledge
2 Park Square, Milton Park, Abingdon, Oxon OX14 4RN

and by Routledge
52 Vanderbilt Avenue, New York, NY 10017

Routledge is an imprint of the Taylor & Francis Group, an informa business

British Library Cataloguing-in-Publication Data
A catalogue record for this book is available from the British Library

Library of Congress Cataloging-in-Publication Data
A catalog record has been requested for this book

ISBN: 978-0-367-49471-1 (hbk)
ISBN: 978-0-367-49470-4 (pbk)
ISBN: 978-1-003-04630-1 (ebk)

DOI: 10.4324/9781003046301

Typeset in Times New Roman
by MPS Limited, Dehradun

Contents

Figures

Tables

Contributors

Alice Ward is an Occupational Therapist with the Anglian Community Enterprise, UK.

Catherine Hayden is an Occupational Therapist with the Sheffield Teaching Hospital NHS Foundation Trust, UK.

Claire Hart is a the Principal Lecturer (Research and Innovation) at Teesside University, UK.

Jodie Brown is an Occupational Therapist with the Sheffield Teaching Hospital NHS Foundation Trust, UK.

Josephine Barnes is an Occupational Therapist with the Lancashire and South Cumbria NHS Foundation Trust, UK.

Julie Bradbury is an Occupational Therapist with the Sheffield Teaching Hospital NHS Foundation Trust, UK.

Kate Halsall is an Occupational Therapist with the Lancashire and South Cumbria NHS Foundation Trust, UK.

Katie Keys is an Occupational Therapist with the Derbyshire Health Care NHS Foundation Trust, UK.

Katrina Reece is an Occupational Therapist with the Derbyshire Healthcare NHS Foundation Trust, UK.

Laura McCafferty is an Occupational Therapist with NHS Grampian, UK.

Laura Murray is an Occupational Therapist with the Anglian Community Enterprise, UK.

Leonie Boland is an Honorary Lecturer in Occupational Therapy at the University of Plymouth, UK.

Lisa Jamieson is an Occupational Therapist with NHS Grampian, UK.

Lorrae Mynard is the Occupational Therapy Educator with Forensicare, Victoria, Australia.

Natalie Jones is the Acting Head Occupational Therapist at the Sheffield Teaching Hospital NHS Foundation Trust, UK.

Polly Blaydes is the Trust AHP Professional Lead and Recovery Services Advisor with the Lincolnshire Partnership NHS Foundation Trust, UK.

Rachel Aiston is an Occupational Therapist with the Sheffield Teaching Hospital NHS Foundation Trust, UK.

Rodrigo Frade is an Occupational Therapist with the Sligo Leitrim Mental Health Services, Ireland.

Samantha Bicker is the Professional Lead for Occupational Therapy at the Inner North Brisbane Mental Health, Australia.

Sharon McMorrow is an Occupational Therapist with the Sligo Leitrim Mental Health Services, Ireland.

Stephanie Glover is an Occupational Therapist with the Lancashire and South Cumbria NHS Foundation Trust, UK.

Theresa Peacock is an Occupational Therapist Manager with the Sligo Leitrim Mental Health Services, Ireland.

Therese Vecsey is an Occupational Therapist with the Derbyshire Healthcare NHS Foundation Trust, UK.

Foreword

The idea of formulation has been present in my practice as an occupational therapist for many years, and I am honoured to have been asked by Sue Parkinson to co-author this exciting new text which I believe will transform Occupational Therapy practice. Like me, some of you will have worked in services where a multidisciplinary case formulation is common. It was during my time working with children and young people with mental health difficulties that I began to wonder what more occupational therapists could offer to the formulation process. However, it was not until I met Sue and started my doctoral research that the notion of occupational formulation began to take shape.

To provide some personal context: when working in mental health services as an occupational therapist I observed the dominance of psychological and medical ways of thinking about people. Although I recognise the value of these ways of thinking, I believe that occupational therapists bring something else - an understanding of someone's occupational life and health through occupation. It was whilst looking to develop greater attention to occupation in my practice that I first encountered Sue. She was running a workshop about the Model of Human Occupation and its assessment tools and inspired me with her knowledge of the model, the depth it brought to her understanding of clients, and the vision it gave to her Occupational Therapy service.

Following Sue's workshop, I was able to use the constructs in the Model of Human Occupation as a framework for my clinical practice. Sue and I remained in contact and we went on to jointly deliver workshops about using the Model of Human Occupation and its assessment tools for Occupational Therapy practice with children, young people, and families. Applying the model in my own work led me to think about how this could be used in formulations. Historically, formulation sat with the clinical psychologists in my team, and this was also reflected in the literature, but I noticed that examples were beginning to emerge of its use by nurses and by social workers too. Then, during my 2015 ethnographic study of occupational therapists in children and young people's mental health (Brooks 2016), I observed occupational therapists contributing their own formulations.

It was during my observation of a team meeting that my research participant was asked to 'go away, complete your assessment and occupational formulation and bring it back to the team'. That occupational therapist was skilled and experienced in using the Model of Human Occupation and its assessments, and used the constructs of this to develop an occupational formulation. Their perspective complemented a psychological formulation and a medical diagnosis.

When writing my research, I realised that Sue was delivering workshops about case formulation and measurable goals for occupational therapists. Sue's understanding of formulation had grown and was driven by her passion, knowledge, and clinical expertise of the Model of Human Occupation. Together, we began to discuss how to develop formulation into a more tangible process for occupational therapists and I invited her to co-write an article on the subject.

We agreed that formulation should become a recognised stage in the Occupational Therapy process, between assessment and goals. I firmly believed that a formulation should be informed by theory and that it provides an important step for occupational therapists to demonstrate theory-informed practice. Sue firmly believed in the collaborative nature of a formulation, and that where possible it should be developed with a client. We both agreed that the nature of Occupational Therapy and formulation lends itself to people's narratives, and whilst our professional expertise lies in applying the theory of occupation, the client brings the expertise to their life story.

Our article became an opinion piece in the British Journal of Occupational Therapy (Brooks and Parkinson 2018) and we have been delighted with the response. It remained in the top ten most-read articles in the journal for some time, and it is one of the highest-scoring journal outputs as measured by Altimetrics. Sue and I have also been thrilled by the personal responses that we have received. Occupational therapists are telling us that formulation gives them a language and a structure to demonstrate their professional reasoning to their team, and supports collaborative goal setting and interventions with clients. We have heard how the paper has been discussed in journal clubs and at team meetings and about occupational therapists who are embedding formulation into their practice.

I am excited to have this opportunity to develop occupational formulation further in this new book. The book is structured sequentially to develop your knowledge and skill. We have paid special attention to making it accessible and useful to practice. The book has three sections each subdivided into chapters. In the first two sections, the chapters provide you with the rationale and theory that underpins the need for formulation and goals. We have included *Author's Notes* to give you examples of application to practise as well as hints and tips. Please also refer to the Tables and Figures which summarise key points. Finally, in Section 3, you will find one of the most important aspects of the book: 20 examples of occupational formulations. Sue reached out to the Occupational Therapy community to develop these examples so that they reflect current practice and the reality of Occupational Therapy today. It is these examples that bring occupational formulation to life.

This book is useful to students who are learning to appreciate the scope of Occupational Therapy, and to novice and experienced clinicians who are keen to hone their professional reasoning skills and to demonstrate their person- and occupation-centred perspective. It will challenge and empower you to change your practice for the better.

Dr Rob Brooks

References

Brooks, R (2016) *Occupational Practice in Children and Young Peoples Mental Health*. PhD Thesis. University of Huddersfield. Available at: http://eprints.hud.ac.uk/id/eprint/30195/ Accessed 01/05/2020.

Brooks R, Parkinson S (2018) Occupational formulation: a three-part structure. *British Journal of Occupational Therapy*, *81*(3), 177-79.

Dr Rob Brooks has worked for over 20 years with children, young people and families with occupational challenges related to physical, mental, and social difficulties. He is the Course Director for Occupational Therapy at Leeds Beckett where his teaching focuses on the use of models in Occupational Therapy practice and his research interests are related to how occupational participation interventions enable health and wellbeing outcomes. He has published and spoken nationally and internationally on a range of topics relating to Occupational Therapy with young people.

Preface

If there is one thing that has characterised my professional life, it has been the desire to communicate complex matters that are of fundamental importance with as much clarity and simplicity as I can manage. I do not suppose that I will ever master this art, and it sometimes seems like an impossible task, but I keep on trying. One of the things that keep me going is knowing that my search has been infinitely enriched and assisted by the work of Gary Kielhofner and the Model of Human Occupation (MOHO) (ed. Taylor 2017). Models are sometimes criticised for oversimplifying life, but MOHO is multi-faceted, intricate, nuanced, and dynamic, and yet still simple enough to have helped me manage the complexity of issues I faced as an occupational therapist, and the challenges experienced on a daily basis by those I worked with.

Gary once paid me the greatest compliment when he described my own work as 'simple'. It seemed to me that he knew the value of simplicity, as well as generosity and integrity. He certainly prized tools that demonstrated a basic utility – not just reliability and validity. Occupational formulation is one such tool – one that has long been associated with the Model of Human Occupation, and which theorists have often linked to the model because of its ability to craft a simple and yet coherent narrative.

I have come to love the way in which a narrative style can pare away the layers of technical analysis to reveal essential truths. For this reason, Rob and I have chosen to include our own stories and viewpoints in this book, in the form of *Author's Notes*, often written using the first person-singular. If you find academic writing a turn-off, then I trust that you will still be able to get a sense of how to create an occupational formulation by reading the *Author's Notes* alone. More than this, my hope is that the example formulations in the last section of the book will express more about Occupational Therapy and the occupational nature of people's lives than we are capable of explaining. In fact, if this is your first introduction to occupational formulation using MOHO, I heartily recommend that you skip straight to the third section and let the stories of people's occupational lives flow over you and through you.

All the stories are fictitious, with the exception of Mr J in the 17th example, and they were composed in collaboration with occupational therapists who recounted their various experiences to me. It was a privilege to listen to their stories and to try to piece together a range of vivid formulations to represent the diversity of occupational life and the typical scope of Occupational Therapy. I cannot pretend that I have achieved this fully. Each story is unique, and in that sense, it cannot represent the vast range of occupations that people participate in. Besides, although I have been lucky enough to work with occupational therapists in Ireland and Australia, I acknowledge that the majority of the examples stem from the UK. That said, I never fail to be impressed when I teach occupational formulation, both by the variety of occupational issues described by the workshop participants and by their common focus as occupational therapists. I hope that the overview of the occupational issues at the end of this book might prompt a similar feeling and inspire you to develop unique, person-centred occupational formulations wherever you work in the world.

Each formulation in this book follows the same pattern – with a beginning, a middle, and an end – to give a sense of a person's occupational identity, occupational competence, and the resulting focus of Occupational Therapy. Meanwhile, the preceding sections have been designed to give you lots of suggestions, hints, and 'top tips' for constructing a well-formed formulation. All the dos and don'ts are meant to be helpful, but please remember that no formulation can replace a therapist's own professional reasoning and therapeutic use of self. Ultimately, these are the factors that will determine the effectiveness of therapy. Similarly, although I am perhaps most proud of my work to make writing measurable occupational goals a reality, I recognise that measurable goals are not essential to good practice. I continue to believe, however, that occupational formulations and measurable occupational goals have the power to enhance the practice of Occupational Therapy. The two are interconnected, with formulations making a case for focusing on three or four issues over the mid- to long-term, and measurable goals articulating the way forward in the short-term.

When you read any of the formulations, ask yourself the following questions. ... Do I get a sense of the person? ... Do I have hope for this person? ... If I had to assume responsibility for the therapy with this person, would I know what needed to be done? If the answers are 'Yes', then the formulation will have served its purpose and will help to support continuity of care, whether or not it is perfectly written. It is almost impossible to write a flawless formulation, especially in a clinical, time-pressured situation, (and I do not claim that the formulations in this book are perfectly written) but with practice, you will get better and better. Supervision can be really helpful too. As a supervisor, I used to read the identity and competence sections and then see if I could guess what the issues would be. Try it! If you can deduce the focus of therapy, then it is a sign that the formulation has made a good case for the issues.

I have lost count of how many occupational therapists have asked me 'Why are we not taught occupational formulation and measurable goals at university?' and for my own part, I often regret that therapists are not taught systematically to apply an evidence-based model in any depth. So I would be delighted if this book goes some way to help occupational therapists and students of Occupational Therapy to appreciate the Model of Human Occupation, and the power of occupational formulation and measurable occupational goals using MOHO.

Sue Parkinson

Reference

Taylor RR ed. (2017) *Kielhofner's Model of Human Occupation*. 5th ed. Philadelphia: Wolters Kluwer.

Sue Parkinson is the lead author of the Model of Human Occupation Screening Tool, (MOHOST) (2006), and the second author of the Model of Human Occupation Exploratory Level Outcome Ratings (MOHO-ExpLOR) (2017). She has worked as a freelance trainer providing workshops in the use of MOHO assessments since 2003 and has also written an intervention programme called Recovery through Activity (2014), which is underpinned by the MOHO framework and aims to promote the long-term benefits of occupational participation.

Acknowledgements

We are deeply grateful to Renée Taylor, editor of Kielhofner's Model of Human Occupation (MOHO) textbook (2017) and director of the MOHO Web, for endorsing this book as a MOHO resource. Our thanks also go to Gail Fisher, lead author of the Residential Environment Impact Scale (2014) and Carmen de las Heras de Pablo, lead author of the Volitional Questionnaire (2007) and the Remotivation Process (2003, 2019,) who have sustained Sue with their loving support and their deep-rooted knowledge of MOHO theory over many years. Most of all, we are indebted to Gary Kielhofner, MOHO's foremost author, who invited Sue to collaborate with him many years ago, on the strength of a single letter that she had sent to him.

Our MOHO journey has been influenced by so many people, and the more that we have taught occupational formulation and measurable occupational goals, the more we have been able to refine our ideas. Thank you to everyone who has added to our understanding, either by offering their insights at a workshop or by sending their work to be reviewed. Particular thanks are due to Derek Raitt, Professional Lead Occupational Therapist at Humber NHS Foundation Trust, for supporting the earliest efforts to write this book and to staff at Leeds Beckett University for their support in the later stages.

In addition, we wish to acknowledge all those who have encouraged us by embedding occupational formulations and goals using MOHO in their practice and to credit the following individuals who have inspired and supported our work.

Carla O'Hara
Occupational Therapist
Sligo Leitrim Mental Health Services, Ireland

Dee Christie
Retired Occupational Therapist, UK
Nice Fellow 2016-2019

Eddie Fenn
Occupational Therapist
Greater Manchester Mental Health NHS
  Foundation Trust, UK

Denise Harper
Retired Specialist Teacher
Derbyshire, UK

Nathalie Daughtry
Occupational Therapist
Sheffield Health and Social Care NHS
  Foundation Trust, UK

Suzie Willis
Allied Health Professional Lead
Camden & Islington NHS Foundation
  Trust, UK

Last but not least, we offer our heartfelt thanks to those who have reviewed the example formulations and/or contributed to the professional perspectives that are included in this book. *A Guide to the Formulation of Plans and Goals in Occupational Therapy* would not have been possible without your collaboration.

References

de las Heras, CG Geist, R Kielhofner, G Li Y (2007) *A User's Guide to the Volitional Questionnaire (VQ), Version 4.1.* Chicago: University of Illinois.

de las Heras CG, Llerana V, Kielhofner G (2003) *A User's Manual for Remotivation Process: Progressive Intervention for Individuals With Severe Volitional Challenges, Version 1.0.* Chicago: University of Illinois at Chicago.

de las Heras CG, Llerana V, Kielhofner G [posthumous] (2019) *The Remotivation Process: Progressive Intervention for Individuals With Severe Volitional Challenges: A User's Manual, Version 2.0.* Chicago: University of Illinois at Chicago.

Fisher G, Forsyth K, Harrison M, Angarolla R, Kayhan E, Noga P, Johnson C, Irvine L (2014) *The Residential Environment Impact Scale, Version 4.0.* Chicago: University of Illinois.

Taylor RR ed. (2017) *Kielhofner's Model of Human Occupation.* 5th ed. Philadelphia: Wolters Kluwer.

Part I

Understanding the concept of a formulation

1 Where does the idea of formulation come from?

A brief history

Case formulation is firmly established in psychotherapy (Eells 2001) and in psychology, where one of the roles of a qualified psychologist is to take a lead on psychological formulation within the team (BPS 2011). It is also beginning to find favour in medicine (Macneil et al. 2012), mental health nursing (Rainforth and Laurenson 2014) and social work (Lee and Toth 2016). It is perhaps more surprising that case formulation has only just begun to be mentioned in occupational therapy literature (Brooks and Parkinson 2018); given that occupational therapists profess that they are not diagnosis-led (Robertson 2012).

Although occupational formulation is in the early stages of development, the foundations have been well-prepared. Back in 1969, the occupational therapist, Line, argued that the case method was a scientific form of clinical thinking, and encouraged the development of 'problem statements'. These statements placed the person's problems

> 'in relation to assets and liabilities in social adaptation, activities of daily living adaptation, and disease adaptation … [supporting] the philosophy that occupational performance may be improved by strengthening assets as well as minimizing liabilities' (Rogers 1982)

By the 1980s, occupational therapists were moving further away from the medical model and were redoubling their efforts to assert their occupational focus with varying degrees of success. Cubie and Kaplan (1982), for example, voiced their concern that many of the clinical decisions made by occupational therapists were based on intuition rather than a consistent reasoning process. They called for a more systematic approach to case analysis, based on the Model of Human Occupation (ed. Taylor 2017), and called for assessment tools to be developed to gather relevant occupational data.

Box 1.1 Author's note

by Sue Parkinson

I first heard about case formulation being used by occupational therapists when listening to Suzie Willis talk about 'Conceptualising clients from standardised assessments' at an Occupational Therapy conference (Willis and Forsyth 2003). A few years later, I was fortunate to be inducted into the same conceptualisation process, as part of a scholarship of practice with the UK

DOI: 10.4324/9781003046301-1

Centre of Outcomes, Research and Education (UKCORE), directed by Kirsty Forsyth, Lynn Summerfield Mann, and Gary Kielhofner (Forsyth et al. 2005a). I began to witness how formulation and measurable goals could transform the therapeutic relationship and occupational therapy outcomes, and by 2010 I was being invited to talk about my experiences with others.

My ideas regarding how to structure formulations and measurable goals have continued to develop over the last decade, and have been shaped by working with hundreds of wonderful occupational therapists, including Lisa Jamieson, who described formulation as the 'key for unlocking potential' (Jamieson and Parkinson 2017).

The Model of Human Occupation (ed. Taylor 2017) now offers a range of formal and informal assessments (Taylor 2017), but difficulties with articulating professional reasoning persist. The prevalence of psychological formulations may even have the power to distract occupational therapists from their occupational focus. For instance, Weiste (2016) was concerned that occupational therapists should focus on more than emotional regulation if they are to offer practical solutions to problems of everyday life, but did not appear to question why occupational therapists were spending their time offering counselling rather than more occupation-based interventions. In her article – *Formulations in Occupational therapy: managing talk about psychiatric outpatients' emotional states* – formulation was viewed simply as an ongoing process of reframing and redirecting a person's focus during a conversation.

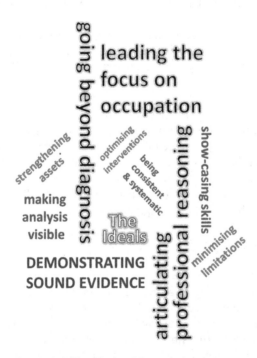

Figure 1.1 The ideals of formulation.

Even when occupational therapy interventions are occupation-based, therapists may not be writing their treatment plans in a way that persuades the reader of its occupational relevance or importance (Page et al. 2015). More specifically, they may be neglecting the importance of their tacit knowledge, and in doing so they risk under-optimising their interventions (Carrier et al. 2010). This is a matter of real concern for theorists and practitioners who are convinced that the core skills of an occupational therapist lie not only in their visible interventions but also in their reasoning skills which are too often invisible – a concern that was articulated by Turner and Alsop (2015):

> '*The challenge for all occupational therapists is to make the invisible reasoning processes visible through the appropriate use of profession-specific language in discourses, assessments, reports, outcome measures, presentations and conversations, so that sound evidence is shown to underpin occupational therapists' visible practice*' (p747)

Occupational formulation provides the ideal platform for showcasing occupational reasoning skills. Connell (2015) goes so far as to recommend that occupational therapists should contribute their unique perspective to an integrated formulation, which she argues is necessary for a multidisciplinary approach in forensic services. This process requires that occupational therapists are able to offer a coherent formulation that others can comprehend in the first place. Thompson (2012) sets out a more ambitious plan, by urging the profession to practise case formulation in all complex cases, allowing their reasons for tailoring interventions to each person to be defined and made transparent. This call has been actively pursued by occupational therapists using the Model of Human Occupation (MOHO) (ed. Taylor 2017). So much so, that formulation is finally being recognised as a vital part of the occupational therapy process (Brooks and Parkinson 2018, Forsyth 2017) which would benefit from having a universal structure (Brooks and Parkinson 2018).

Box 1.2   Author's note

by Sue Parkinson

I would not be recommending the process of occupational formulation if I did not have experience of its feasibility and effectiveness across a range of occupational therapy services. Much of this experience stems from having worked as a Practice Development Advisor for occupational therapists in a large healthcare organisation in the UK, where MOHO had been adopted and occupational formulation had been introduced. A service-wide audit demonstrated that the vast majority of my occupational therapy colleagues were able to meet our agreed standards for occupational formulation, and a later survey indicated that it was possible for formulations to be documented in the majority of occupational therapy case notes (unpublished data).

The organisation in which I worked provided services for mental health and learning disability, and had facilities for children, adults, and older adults in community and inpatient settings. The only services struggling to document fully-developed formulations were those in fast-paced acute settings with high caseload turnovers. Even here, however, occupational therapists were able to verbalise the outlines of formulations, produce succinct summaries and proceed to negotiate measurable goals based on the long-term issues identified, rather than short-term aims. Given that my clinical work was predominantly in acute mental health, this outcome continues to inspire me. I have always believed that inpatient settings offer more than short-term relief, and I am thrilled that even the most rudimentary of occupational formulations can pave the way for a person's recovery journey as they transition into the community.

In more recent years, I have explored the potential for occupational formulation with occupational therapists working in physical services, where occupation-centred practice has proved to be a challenge. It has been heartening to see how occupational formulation can offer the prospect of countering a process-led culture, and allow therapists to demonstrate their ability to be truly person-centred. These encounters have led me to agree wholeheartedly with Rob Brooks in endorsing the occupational formulation process across the breadth of occupational therapy practice (Parkinson and Brooks 2018).

References

Brooks R, Parkinson S (2018) Occupational formulation: a three-part structure. *British Journal of Occupational Therapy*, *81(3)*, 177–179.

Carrier A, Levasseur M, Bédard D, Desrosiers J (2010) Community occupational therapists' clinical reasoning: identifying tacit knowledge. *Australian Occupational Therapy Journal*, *57(6)*, 356–365.

Connell C (2015) An integrated case formulation approach in forensic practice: the contribution of occupational therapy to risk assessment and formulation. *The Journal of Forensic Psychiatry and Psychology*, *26(1)*, 94–106.

Cubie SH, Kaplan K (1982) A case analysis method for the Model of Human Occupation. *American Journal of Occupational Therapy*, *36(10)*, 645–656.

Eells T (2001) Update on psychotherapy case formulation research. *The Journal of Psychotherapy Practice and Research*, *10(4)*, 277–281.

Forsyth K (2017) Therapeutic reasoning: planning, implementing, and evaluating the outcomes of therapy. In: RR Taylor ed. *Kielhofner's Model of Human Occupation: Theory and Application*. Philadelphia: Wolters Kluwer. 159–172.

Forsyth K, Mann LS, Kielhofner G (2005a) Scholarship of practice: making occupation-focused, theory-driven, evidence-based practice a reality. *British Journal of Occupational Therapy*, *68(6)*, 260–267.

Jamieson L, Parkinson S (2017) Unlocking potential: case formulation and measurable goals in a prison setting. *Occupational Therapy News*, *25(3)*, 36–38.

Lee E, Toth H (2016) An integrated case formulation in social work. Towards developing a theory of a client. *Smith College Studies in Social Work*, *86(3)*, 184–203.

Macneil CA, Hasty MK, Conus P, Berk M (2012) Is diagnosis enough to guide interventions in mental health? Using case formulation in clinical practice. *BMC Medicine, 10*, 111. DOI: 10. 1186/1741-7015-10-111. Accessed 08/08/2019.

Page J, Roos K, Bänziger A, Margot-Cattin I, Agustoni S, Rossini E, Meichtry A, Meyer S (2015) Formulating goals in occupational therapy: state of the art in Switzerland. *Scandinavian Journal of Occupational Therapy*, *22(6)*, 403–15.

Rainforth M, Laurenson M (2014) A literature review of case formulation to inform mental health practice. *Journal of Psychiatric and Mental Health Nursing, 21(3)*, 206–13.

Robertson L (2012) *Clinical Reasoning in Occupational Therapy: Controversies in Practice.* Chichester: John Wiley and Sons.

Rogers JC (1982) Order and disorder in Occupational Therapy. *American Journal of Occupational Therapy, 36(1)*, 29–35.

Taylor RR ed. (2017) *Kielhofner's Model of Human Occupation.* 5th ed. Philadelphia: Wolters Kluwer.

Taylor RR, Kielhofner G [posthumous] (2017) Introduction to the Model of Human Occupation. In: RR Taylor ed. *Kielhofner's Model of Human Occupation.* 5th ed. Philadelphia: Wolters Kluwer. 3–10.

Thompson BF (2012) Abductive reasoning and case formulation in complex cases. In: L Robertson ed. *Clinical Reasoning in Occupational Therapy.* Pondicherry: Wiley-Blackwell. 15–30.

Turner A, Alsop A (2015) Unique core skills: exploring occupational therapists' hidden assets. *British Journal of Occupational Therapy, 78(12)*, 739–749.

Weiste E (2016) Formulations in occupational therapy: managing talk about psychiatric out-patients' emotional states. *Journal of Pragmatics, 105*, 59–73.

Willis S, Forsyth K (2003) Conceptualising clients from standardised assessments. *Design for Living Life: College of Occupational Therapists, 27th annual conference and exhibition.* Glasgow: College of Occupational Therapists.

2 What is a formulation?

A formulation, or a *case* formulation as it is commonly known, is grounded in assessment and provides the basis for making decisions about the way ahead (British Psychological Society [BPS] 2011). It attempts to make sense of the rich and varied information gleaned during the course of assessment by pulling all the relevant strands into a coherent whole so that treatment plans and goals can be negotiated clearly and openly. A single assessment may not result in the appropriate depth and breadth of comprehension, thus, the formulation is not attempted until the initial assessment *phase* is concluded. Until this time, the clinician and the client might agree on a number of general aims which can be refined once the important issues emerge and are better understood.

Once clinicians start to get a sense of the way forward, they must share their ideas with their clients as much as possible and continue to work in close partnership as the formulation takes shape. Draft formulations should also be discussed with key others and gauged in relation to professional opinion so those insights can be shared and hypotheses can be tested (Kuyken 2006) (see Figure 2.1). In doing so, clinicians seek to strengthen their reasoning and obtain support or validation for their unique contribution, enabling interventions to be prioritised and desired outcomes to be agreed (BPS 2011).

Box 2.1 Author's note

by Dr Rob Brooks

It is my belief that assessments provide little benefit unless they inform the treatment process, and that assessment results become more relevant when they contribute to a formulation which explains the person's circumstances rather than simply listing the person's strengths and limitations. The assessment information benefits from being organised into a cohesive framework that includes only the most relevant findings, and highlights key issues while conveying acute respect for the person's unique situation. For me, the Model of Human Occupation (ed. Taylor 2017) has always supported this process, by articulating how personal characteristics and the environment interact with each other to influence occupational adaptation (Parkinson et al. 2008).

Occupational formulation is a reflective process that synthesises rich information and requires in-depth occupational therapy assessment. It will draw upon the values and goals of the person, their appraisal of their own

---

DOI: 10.4324/9781003046301-2

ability, and their expectation of success in the future. Interestingly, however, when I teach occupational formulation, it is not uncommon for students and therapists to realise that their assessment to date has been insufficient. In their rush to assess a person's competence in basic tasks, they may not be fully aware of the person's subjective viewpoint or they may not have gathered any information about how the person performs valued activities. The formulation process fosters pronounced thoughtfulness and reflection, and my hope is that it will stimulate a more holistic assessment process.

Reading through the diverse definitions for formulations, it is easy to lose sight of its key components. Yet in one form or another, most definitions refer to a combination of three processes:

- collaboration
- contextualisation
- conceptualisation

Taking this a stage further, it might be said that a case formulation communicates clinical reasoning by:

- collaborating with the person to convey a shared or co-created understanding
- contextualising the key contributory factors to aid comprehension
- conceptualising complex needs to establish a case for intervention

Collaboration

Hypotheses are likely to be more robust when they are agreed in partnership with others and tested with all those involved. Accordingly, mutual sharing and collaboration are viewed as the hallmarks of effective therapy (Thompson 2012), and case formulation is rooted in shared understanding (Macneil et al. 2012) and meaning-making (Statewide Behaviour Intervention Service [SBIS] 2017) between the therapist and

- the service user
- carers
- the team
- other professional agencies

First and foremost, formulations must involve the individual service user to the greatest extent possible (Forsyth 2017). Ideally, this will eliminate any notion of the therapist being the expert and engage service users as equals (SBIS 2017). Ultimately, it may even allow individuals to become self-directed (SBIS 2017) – essentially becoming their own therapists, (Thompson 2012). It will certainly strengthen the therapeutic relationship (*ibid*) by involving individuals in decision-making (Rainforth and Laurenson 2014) and by blending the knowledge of professionals with the lived experiences of service users (Henderson and Martin 2014).

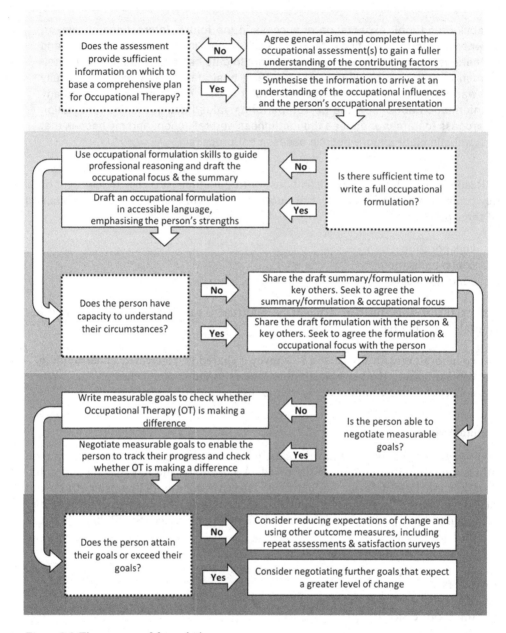

Figure 2.1 The process of formulation.

At the very least, when collaboration is challenged by the reduced capacity of the individual, who may be living with advanced dementia, or a severe brain injury, or profound learning disabilities, the therapist should take account of the person's preferred way of doing things (Kuyken 2006) and aim to identify distinctive aspects of their presentation (Macneil et al. 2012). Collaboration with carers becomes all the more important in these circumstances, especially when the eventual goals might include the reduction of carer burden or assistance. In these circumstances, the intentions of the formulation would be to help carers feel understood, and to pave the way for any joint working with the therapist in the future.

Similarly, opportunities for teamwork are maximised by communicating the case formulation to the multidisciplinary team. In doing so, the therapist supports everyone to be clearer about the person's goals (Thompson 2012) and promotes a shared understanding (BPS 2011). This might lead to goals being held in common across the team (SBIS 2017) and a shared agenda being developed, allowing interventions to be targeted with greater consistency (Macneil et al. 2012).

Finally, a case formulation document makes an invaluable record to share with other professional agencies such as hostels, schools, care homes, and courts (BPS 2011). It encourages the seamless transfer of care by providing a voice for the person and reporting information in a way that is positive, respectful, and sensitive (SBIS 2017).

> **Box 2.2   Author's note**
>
> *by Sue Parkinson*
>
> While it is true that a written formulation may not be co-authored by the individual concerned, the formulation is a culmination of a consultative process and aims to integrate the person's perspective. When it is shared or recounted, the person should be able to recognise themselves and feel listened to, and they should be able to acknowledge any objective descriptions recorded by the therapist. They should be offered the opportunity to agree with the formulation and this may involve tweaking the wording to arrive at the most accurate interpretation of events. In this way, the most sensitive formulations will reveal whether a person's subjective viewpoints correspond with objective reality and gently challenge any preconceived ideas held by those who are contributing to it.
>
> I have heard of countless examples when occupational formulation has been pivotal in creating a shared understanding, and where the therapist and client have refined the original formulation to the person's satisfaction. I have even heard of one instance when a person – a teacher by profession – took out his red marking pen to make amendments. This was welcomed by the therapist, as it showed that the formulation was worth amending and allowed the person to truly own his formulation.

Contextualisation

Thompson (2012) recognises that the process of formulation is not straightforward and contends that this process relies on abductive reasoning. She states that:

> 'Abductive reasoning involves working from descriptions of patterns to possible explanations for those patterns. It differs from deduction because it works from patterns to explanations that are *most likely* rather than from patterns to the *only explanation,* and it differs from induction because it works from *patterns* to explanations rather than from *individual pieces of information* to some sort of general rule' (p19)

A case formulation does not, therefore, consist of a mere list of individual factors that contribute to an individual's ongoing presentation. The factors need to be placed in context in order to make a convincing case for intervention – one which sheds light on patterns of behaviours, and transforms multiple assessment findings to allow the 'whole picture' to emerge (Pierre and Sonn 1999); furthermore, one which enables diverse information to be distilled into a concise account (Hart et al. 2011).

The process of contextualisation involves comparing and contrasting a range of factors so that:

- limitations are viewed in the context of a person's strengths (Macneil et al. 2012, Thompson 2012, Brooks and Parkinson 2018)
- the person is viewed in the context of their environment (SBIS 2017) including their socio-cultural environment (BPS 2011)
- the person's subjective experience is viewed in the context of their observed performance (Brooks and Parkinson 2018)
- current performance is viewed in the context of personal history, including previous traumas (BPS 2011) and changes to personal circumstances (Lee and Kielhofner [posthumous] 2017)
- presenting issues are viewed in the context of clinical knowledge and theory (SBIS 2017)

In the same way that each person has strengths and limitations, the environment also provides opportunities and resources, as well as demands and constraints (Fisher et al. 2017). Placing any findings in the context of the environment will increase objectivity and supports realistic decision-making. The desires of the person will be balanced with the constraints of the environment (Thompson 2012); the impact of the physical environment on the person's skills will be identified (Cubie and Kaplan 1982); and the influence of the person's social and cultural background will be acknowledged (Rainworth and Laurenson 2014).

In addition to recognising the importance of environmental considerations, the formulation also needs to present the person's subjective viewpoint and feelings alongside any empirical observations (Brooks and Parkinson 2018). The therapist's underlying philosophy and theoretical understanding will then provide a secure foundation from which the presenting issues and interventions emerge. They provide a cohesive structure that brings ideas together (Henderson and Martin 2014), pulling together disparate facts to create a set of arguments that represent the professional's unique perspective (Forsyth 2017). A psychological formulation is therefore grounded in psychological theory and evidence (BPS 2011) while an occupational formulation draws naturally on occupational frameworks/models and focuses on occupational issues related to self-care, productivity, and leisure (Parkinson et al. 2008, 2011).

Box 2.3   Author's note

by Dr Rob Brooks

A formulation is based on the understanding that multiple factors must be grasped if you are to arrive at a true understanding. If you put a person's performance into context, it shows that you appreciate where the person is coming from – the battles and trials they have faced, as well as the hopes and dreams that they have. In doing so, you send a strong, two-fold message that the presenting problems are not being attributed to personal faults but to a dynamic interaction with external forces and that the person has strengths that can be built upon.

Emphasising a person's strengths is particularly important because it is essential that hope is cultivated if a formulation is to provide compelling reasons for therapy. It is all too easy for the clinical team to focus on the presenting problems – the reasons for intervening – rather than the assets that are part of the solution. Occupational therapists need to resist this tendency in order to play a key role in Remotivation (de las Heras de Pablo et al. 2019) and promoting hope when an individual feels hopeless. Thus, being able to identify and articulate the person's strengths is crucial.

This does not mean that a person's limitations should be ignored, instead, they should be viewed in parallel with the capabilities that a person has. It is not a case of creating a false picture, but of simply emphasising strengths and refraining from judging or catastrophizing any limitations. In doing so, I believe that occupational therapists can offer an alternative sense of the occupational influences and the person's occupational presentation that the person can recognise and embrace. The purpose is to remain true to the person's understanding of their own lives while shifting their narrative to one of hope and recovery.

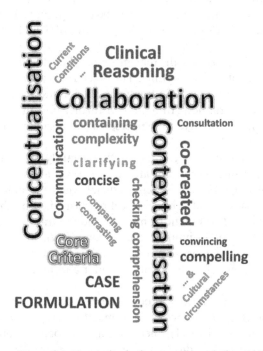

Figure 2.2 Core criteria for case formulation (All the C's).

Conceptualisation

Essentially, a case formulation is a hypothesis (BPS 2011) or a way of making sense of information (Forsyth 2017) which 'represents the clinician's best thinking' about the dynamics affecting a person (SBIS 2017). It aims to generate an explanatory theory regarding the factors that precipitate and maintain a person's specific needs (Robertson 2012), by "identifying individualised contributing factors and how these could influence the person's presentation" (Macneil et al. 2012, p1).

Proponents of case formulation assert that medical diagnosis alone is an insufficient guide for intervention-planning (Macneil et al. 2012, Robertson 2012). They proposed that case formulation may fill the 'explanatory gap' between diagnosis and treatment (Eells 2001). Furthermore, it fills a gap between *assessment* and treatment, and has been described as 'a bridge between the assessment and treatment phases' (Rainforth and Laurenson 2014, p206). It can therefore help occupational therapists to 'create an understanding of what the assessment information is telling them ... and guide the next step' (Forsyth 2017, p164).

The next step can broadly be defined in terms of intervention-planning, including the development of measurable goals (Parkinson et al. 2011, Forsyth 2017). The formulation guides and informs possible intervention (BPS 2011) by helping clinicians to select, prioritise, and design specific interventions (Hart et al. 2011, Macneil et al. 2012, SBIS 2017) leading to the development of individualised treatment options (Robertson 2012). On the other hand,

> 'Formulation does not necessarily lead to intervention; it may indicate that no further input from professionals is needed. It should also be noted that developing a formulation can be a powerful intervention in itself, and may be enough on its own to enable the service user or team to move forward and make changes' (BPS 2011, p9)

When interventions are recommended, it is worth remembering that these are only provisional (SBIS 2017) and can be altered at anytime. The objective is always to address the person's issues and never to insist on certain treatment modalities. Indeed, it may even be necessary to reformulate a situation (BPS 2011) if further information should come to light, or there are significant changes to the person's circumstances, or progress exceeds initial expectations.

In truth, it is recognised that a person's story is complex and constantly evolving (BPS 2011), but this does not mean that one should not attempt to create a working hypothesis. Rather, formulation should be viewed as being crucial when presented with intricate situations in which clinicians might otherwise feel overwhelmed by the amount of information (Thompson 2012). Formulations mitigate the natural human tendency to be distracted by small details, or to jump to conclusions (*ibid*). Instead, they encourage therapists to reflect on the most important findings (Loftus and Higgs 2008) which will reveal the uniqueness of each person and offer a rationale that illuminates their world.

Clinical reflection could remain as an introspective process, albeit one that draws on and is enhanced by communication with others. However, formulation may become an 'event' (BPS 2011) or a 'product' (Hart et al. 2011) when meetings or consultations are arranged to develop a shared formulation and/or a written account is produced. Understandably, given the fast pace of many services and the time required to facilitate a collaborative endeavour, documenting a formulation may not actually happen until after treatment has started (Thompson 2012), but this does not detract from its value. It still provides an important opportunity to clarify working hypotheses, to review treatment in the early stages, and to turn general aims into specific goals.

Box 2.4   Author's note

by Sue Parkinson

For many years, my assessments highlighted the occupational needs of the people I worked with, and my assessment findings contributed to and complemented the multidisciplinary assessments of each person's history, their symptoms, and general presentation. I became adept at communicating the impact of volition (motivation for occupation), habituation (pattern of occupation), performance, and the environment, but my efforts to explain the therapeutic value of a person participating in everyday occupation were sometimes less successful. I very much regret that I had not learned about, or even heard about, occupational formulation when I was still practising as a clinician.

As a professional advisor and trainer, I am convinced that occupational formulation can serve to counter and complement the prevailing medical model and the psychological approaches which are so pervasive. In my perspective, occupational formulations provide the missing link between the theoretical concepts that aid a deeper understanding of a person's needs, and the practical occupational domains of self-care, productivity, and leisure that characterise the person's life and form the basis for occupational therapy interventions. As such, they are vital for the continuity of care … or in this case, the continuity of *therapy*.

If you have ever stepped in to manage a caseload when another therapist has left, then you will know how difficult it is to get to know the people referred to you without asking them the same questions they have been asked before. You may be able to gain an understanding of the factors influencing a person's presentation by looking at past assessments, but this information does not always help you to understand why certain interventions have been chosen and not others. A formulation, especially if accompanied by measured goals, can fill the gaps in your knowledge and help make the transition as smooth and as seamless as possible.

References

British Psychological Society [BPS] (2011) *Good practice guidelines on the use of psychological formulation*. Leicester: BPS.

Brooks R, Parkinson S (2018) Occupational formulation: a three-part structure. *British Journal of Occupational Therapy*, *81*(3), 177–79.

Cubie SH, Kaplan K (1982) A case analysis method for the Model of Human Occupation. *American Journal of Occupational Therapy*, *36*(10), 645–56.

de las Heras CG, Llerana V, Kielhofner G [posthumous] (2019) *The Remotivation Process: Progressive intervention for individuals with severe volitional challenges: a user's manual. Version 2.0*. Chicago: University of Illinois at Chicago.

Eells T (2001) Update on psychotherapy case formulation research. *The Journal of Psychotherapy Practice and Research*, *10*(4), 277–81.

Fisher G, Parkinson S, Haglund L (2017) The environment and human occupation. In: RR Taylor ed. *Kielhofner's Model of Human Occupation*. 5th ed. Wolters Kluwer, Philadelphia, 91–106.

Forsyth K (2017) Therapeutic reasoning: planning, implementing, and evaluating the outcomes of therapy. In: RR Taylor ed. *Kielhofner's Model of Human Occupation: Theory and Application*. Philadelphia: Wolters Kluwer. 159–72.

Hart S, Sturmey P, Logan C, McMurran M (2011) Forensic case formulation. *International Journal of Forensic Mental Health*, *10(2)*, 118–26.

Henderson SW, Andrés Martin (2014) Case formulation and integration of information in child and adolescent mental health. In: JM Rey ed. *IACAPAP e-Textbook of Child and Adolescent Mental Health*. Geneva: International Association for Child and Adolescent Psychiatry and Allied Professions.

Kuyken W (2006) Evidence-based case formulation: is the emperor clothed? In: N Tarrier ed. *Case Formulation in Cognitive Behaviour Therapy: The Treatment of Challenging and Complex Cases*. Hove, Sussex: Routledge. 12–35.

Lee SW, Kielhofner G [posthumous] (2017) Habituation: patterns of daily occupation. In: RR Taylor ed. *Kielhofner's Model of Human Occupation: Theory and Application*. Philadelphia: Wolters Kluwer. 57–73.

Loftus S, Higgs J (2008) Learning the language of clinical reasoning. In: J Higgs, MA Jones, S Loftus, N Christensen eds. *Clinical Reasoning in the Health Professions*. 3rd ed. Oxford: Butterworth-Heinemann, 399–448.

Macneil CA, Hasty MK, Conus P, Berk M (2012) Is diagnosis enough to guide interventions in mental health? Using case formulation in clinical practice. *BMC Medicine, 10*, 111 DOI: 10.1186/1741-7015-10-111. Accessed 08/08/2019.

Parkinson S, Chester A, Cratchley S, Rowbottom J (2008) Application of the Model of Human Occupation Screening Tool (MOHOST assessment) in an acute psychiatric setting. *Occupational Therapy in Health Care*, *22(2–3)*, 63–75.

Parkinson S, Shenfield M, Reece K, Elliott J (2011) Enhancing clinical reasoning through the use of evidence-based assessments, robust case formulations and measurable goals. *British Journal of Occupational Therapy 74(3)*, 148–152.

Pierre BL, Sonn U (1999) Occupational therapy as documented in patients' records Part I. A content analysis of occupational therapy records at an occupational therapy department. *Scandinavian Journal of Occupational Therapy*, *3(2)*, 79–89.

Rainforth M, Laurenson M (2014) A literature review of case formulation to inform mental health practice. *Journal of Psychiatric and Mental Health Nursing*, *21(3)*, 206–213.

Robertson L (2012). *Clinical Reasoning in Occupational Therapy: Controversies in Practice*. Etobicoke: John Wiley and Sons.

Statewide Behaviour Intervention Service [SBIS] (2017) *Clinical Formulation Practice Guide: A collaborative approach*. Parramatta, Australia: Clinical Innovation and Governance, Ageing, Disability and Home Care, Department of Family and Community Services.

Taylor RR ed. (2017) *Kielhofner's Model of Human Occupation*. 5th ed. Philadelphia: Wolters Kluwer.

Thompson BF (2012) Abductive reasoning and case formulation in complex cases. In: L Robertson ed. *Clinical Reasoning in Occupational Therapy*. Pondicherry: Wiley-Blackwell. 15–30.

3   Why create a formulation?

There would be no point in producing a formulation if the individual is not the primary beneficiary. First and foremost, a formulation should aim to benefit the person and his or her carers and any other benefits should be regarded as secondary, albeit that they make their own indirect contribution to the overall benefit of the person. When taking all the benefits into account, the best formulations will:

*   benefit the person and carers
*   enhance the therapeutic relationship
*   assist the therapist
*   inform the wider team

Benefiting the person and carers

The formulation exists to provide a voice for the person (and carers), and as such it upholds 'the rights, dignity, and safety of the person with disability, their family and services at each stage of the process' (Statewide Behaviour Intervention Service [SBIS] 2017, p15). This involves ensuring that the person's cultural needs are included, emphasising the person's strengths, and normalising problems so that the person and any carers are less prone to blame themselves and more likely to feel both understood and collected (British Psychological Society [BPS] 2011). By acknowledging the strengths of the person and their situation, the process supports the sharing of information in a manner that is positive, respectful, and sensitive (SBIS 2017), and gives meaning and hope to the person and their carers (BPS 2011). In addition, by building on the person's strengths and motivation, the formulation can lead to an improved sense of agency – enabling individuals to exercise control in their preferred ways of making changes (Kuyken 2006).

> **Box 3.1   Author's note**
>
> *by Sue Parkinson*
>
>   In 2008, my colleagues and I wrote an article in which we shared the value of occupational formulation and illustrated the benefits by presenting a single anonymised case study. This described the progress of a woman who had experienced multiple role losses and was left feeling angry and depressed. She had consistently doubted the purpose of occupational therapy, but felt

DOI: 10.4324/9781003046301-3

validated by the occupational formulation. It helped her to place her emotions in context, and she went on to re-engage in her valued occupations (Parkinson et al. 2008).

In 2015, we published a study that indicated that profession-specific practice, including an increased use of formulations and measurable goals, was associated with better occupational outcomes for whole caseloads. It was found that when the practice of occupational therapists was more profession-specific, clients were significantly more satisfied with their ability to complete home-based activities for daily living, and that they reported spending additional time at significantly more community-based locations since their therapy had started. Naturally, multiple factors may have influenced the services that were compared, but we considered that the gains were partly due to profession-specific processes boosting profession-specific reasoning (Parkinson et al. 2015).

In essence, the formulation is a blueprint for a more personalised approach and has the potential for better clinical outcomes for the person (Macneil et al. 2012). Not only does it provide a true account of the person's subjective viewpoint, but it simultaneously helps the person to make sense of their situation and to recognise the value and purpose of therapy (Thompson 2012). Formulations are therefore associated with increased motivation and persistence (Weiste 2016), and may ultimately lead to individuals becoming self-directed (SBIS 2017) by revealing how they might become their own therapists (Thompson 2012).

Enhancing the therapeutic relationship

Studies of occupational therapists mirror previous findings in the field of psychology in suggesting that the relationship between the person and the therapist is the single most important factor influencing the outcome of treatment (Taylor 2008). Demonstrating empathy by formulating the person's own story provides an opportunity for this partnership to be strengthened, and there is emerging evidence that the formulation process is associated with clinicians having more favourable perceptions of the therapeutic relationship (Weiste 2016). This may be because the collaborative nature of formulation strengthens the therapeutic alliance with the person and/or carers (BPS 2011) by providing an opportunity for the sharing of information, mutual reflection, and reciprocal decision-making (SBIS 2017).

A common understanding of the issues and shared meaning-making can be developed through the formulation process, in which participants are encouraged to learn from and about each other and generate fresh ways of thinking about a situation (SBIS 2017). With the person contributing their own experiences and the therapist offering a perception of the contributing factors, there is the exciting potential to gain new insights that neither of them originally held (Forsyth 2017). Although the care required for arriving at a sensitive formulation undoubtedly takes time, this time is well spent. It decreases the likelihood of people having preconceptions or jumping to conclusions (Thompson 2012), thus enabling both parties to have a united vision of what the future could look like.

Box 3.2 Author's note

by Sue Parkinson

To perceive that the formulation enhances the therapeutic alliance and helps to strengthen collaborative work is gratifying, but to have individuals confirm that it created an opportunity to feel understood is even more rewarding. For this reason, my colleagues and I actively sought the opinions of the people that we worked with by conducting a satisfaction survey. This survey, along with another conducted by Lisa Jamieson in prison services, confirmed that individuals viewed occupational formulation as a positive intervention in its own right (Parkinson et al. 2011, Jamieson and Parkinson 2017). To paraphrase some of the statements that they made:

- it helped them to gain a sense of direction
- it helped them to feel that they were being treated as individuals
- it helped them to understand what Occupational Therapy was all about
- it helped them to articulate their own needs

Assisting the therapist

The formulation process supports therapists in clarifying hypotheses (BPS 2011) while remaining open to different viewpoints and appreciating a person's motivations (SBIS 2017). As a consequence, therapists may find that they have developed a deeper understanding of the person (Macneil et al. 2012) and a clearer comprehension of how issues should be targeted and actions might be planned (Richmond 2017). Crafting the formulation will also help any gaps in assessment information to be noticed and

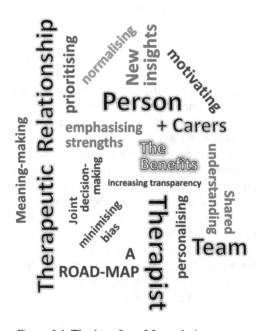

Figure 3.1 The benefits of formulation.

biases in decision-making to be minimised. Pulido-Castelblanco and Gómez (2014) concurred with Eells (2001) when they wrote that,

> *'... case formulation improves the clinical judgment to such an extent that decisions are not based on the therapist's intuition, but on the relations identified for the particular case, which have been explored from a careful assessment of the motive for consultation and problems of the client. This consequently leads to a decrease in that the likelihood of standardised, inefficient, or ambiguous interventions will be done [sic]'* (as translated from Spanish) (p188).

The resulting formulation assists therapists in explaining and focusing their interventions by linking information about the person and theoretical concepts to practical actions. It enables them to organise large amounts of complex information (Kuyken 2006) by taking all the diverse assessment information that they have gathered and bringing it together to form a coherent set of arguments capable of articulating their unique perspective (Forsyth 2017). In effect, they produce a tool that is their constant guide – a tool which Richmond (2017) calls a 'compass' and which Thompson (2012) likens to a 'roadmap' – a means of keeping on track or maintaining direction that reduces the risk of getting lost or being diverted in a maze of interventions.

Robust formulation helps prioritise issues and problems, which in turn will guide the selection and planning of the most effective interventions, and may also identify possible reasons for any future deterioration by noting any responses to interventions and behaviours which might hinder progress (Kuyken 2006, BPS 2011). This helps therapists feel contained (BPS 2011) and more confident in their work, since formulations can provide the basis for excellent ongoing clinical supervision (Kuyken 2006). The supervision process might otherwise lack a shared focus or an agreed structure (Fitzpatrick et al. 2015), and case formulation can offer a format that is more 'scientific' (Page et al. 2008), in that it is methodical, logical, and controlled.

Box 3.3   Author's note

by Sue Parkinson

Having taught occupational formulation for more than a decade, I am constantly delighted when therapists tell me that that such training has helped them to assert their unique professional perspective. This has long been a concern of mine, and I know from first-hand experience how professional development initiatives can strengthen practice by helping therapists to feel valued and by boosting their confidence, and how the Model of Human Occupation (ed. Taylor 2017) can provide a foundation for occupation-focused practice (Parkinson et al. 2010) and occupation-centred therapy.

It is true that therapists may express initial apprehension about the time it takes to produce an occupational formulation, but the overall feeling of so many therapists that I have worked with is that it adds to their understanding of a person's occupational needs. It seems to help clarify issues by providing a logical structure for ordering their thoughts, 'pulling information together' so that all the relevant information can be summarised in one place, consequently giving them greater confidence in articulating the value of their interventions (Parkinson et al. 2011).

Informing the wider team

By simply creating a formulation, a therapist expects to improve the efficacy of their intervention (Carrier et al. 2010), which in turn lessens the burden of care for the whole team. Furthermore, by making the reasoning for the therapist's interventions more transparent, it allows everyone who is involved in providing treatment to have a clearer sense of the goals of therapy (Thompson 2012). As a result, the team may also gain a better understanding of how to support these goals, especially when a comprehensive formulation and treatment plan indicates 'purpose, roles, responsibilities, safety, and boundaries' (SBIS 2017, p15).

Therapists may also facilitate or contribute to formulation meetings which clinicians are known to perceive as being helpful, in part because they feel listened to and in part because they result in a more consistent team approach and have even been linked to increased empathy towards the person (Whitton et al. 2016). Such meetings encourage open discussion, help to create workable hypotheses, and should lead to the generation of system-wide interventions that are in the best interests of the person and their carers (SBIS 2017).

Connell (2015) affirms the advantages of a multi-disciplinary approach to case formulation in forensic practice, where a team approach is vital for risk management. In order to contribute their clinical expertise, occupational therapists should first, of course, be able to formulate their own unique perspective. Doing so will not merely result in short-term gains but could even influence long-term cultural change in which the contribution of the profession is recognised and respected (BPS 2011). This is because a formulation is essentially a case study that captures real experiences and stories that are highly valued, being so much easier to understand than more formal, science-based reports (Korjonen et al. 2016).

Box 3.4   Author's note

by Sue Parkinson

A formulation should help everyone involved to 'understand the rich complexity of occupational behaviour" (Hagedorn, 2000, p63), and a survey conducted by my colleagues found evidence that this was the case (Parkinson et al. 2011).

- Nursing staff valued receiving the 'expert' opinion of an occupational therapist because it helped the whole service to produce 'robust' care plans and 'comprehensive' care packages. They appreciated the skills of the occupational therapists in generating formulations that were 'informative' and 'thorough' while still being 'concise' and 'easy' to understand

- Social Workers recognised that occupational formulations informed their own decisions and enabled them to advocate successfully for people's needs

- Psychologists acknowledged that the occupational formulations complemented their own psychological formulations rather than competing with them. Indeed, the occupational formulations were viewed as being 'vital' for 'effective and joined-up' packages of care

A note of caution

Formulation should not be viewed as a panacea. Even though it has been described as 'the lynchpin that holds theory and practice together' (Butler 1998), Kuyken (2006) questions the validity of such claims and points out that the evidence for formulation, although promising, is limited. He calls for more research and in the meantime sets out criteria by which therapists may determine the relative evidence-base of their formulations. These are divided into top-down criteria (does empirical research underpin the guiding theoretical framework?) and bottom-up criteria (is the process reliable, meaningful, respected, and consistent with other valid measures, and does it improve clinical and cost-effectiveness?).

Improving efficacy is by no means assured. Macneil et al. (2012) report that while many people respond to formulations with increased hope and understanding, some have described negative consequences such as anxiety. They stress the importance of collaboration when developing formulations, the inclusion of strengths, and the need to proceed with sensitivity. They also note that training – even brief training – and ongoing experience have both been consistently associated with improvements in the quality of cognitive behavioural and psychodynamic formulations.

Effective training programmes and supervision may help to guard against the inevitable biases which result from the therapists' own values and beliefs in addition to external influences and expectations (SBIS 2017). Even so, further research will be required to measure the efficacy of such support (Rainforth and Laurenson 2014). Ultimately, case formulations are like case studies in that these are known to vary in quality and content, but they are also likely to benefit from having guidelines and templates to improve their replicability (Korjonen et al. 2016). Bearing this in mind, this book aims to provide a template based on an evidence-based conceptual model of practice, as well as guidelines or 'top tips' to strengthen the practice of occupational formulation.

References

British Psychological Society [BPS] (2011) *Good Practice Guidelines on the Use of Psychological Formulation*. Leicester: BPS.

Butler (1998) Clinical formulation. In: AS Bellack and M Hersen eds. *Comprehensive Clinical Psychology*. New York: Pergammon Press.

Carrier A, Levasseur M, Bédard D, Desrosiers J (2010) Community occupational therapists' clinical reasoning: identifying tacit knowledge. *Australian Occupational Therapy Journal*, *57(6)*, 356–365.

Connell C (2015) An integrated case formulation approach in forensic practice: the contribution of occupational therapy to risk assessment and formulation. *The Journal of Forensic Psychiatry and Psychology*, *26(1)*, 94–106.

Eells T (2001) Update on psychotherapy case formulation research. *The Journal of Psychotherapy Practice and Research*, *10(4)*, 277–281.

Fitzpatrick S, Smith M, Wilding C (2015) Clinical supervision in Allied Health in Australia: a model of allied health clinical supervision based on practitioner experience. *Internet Journal of Allied Health Sciences and Practice*, *13(4)*. Accessed 08/08/2019.

Forsyth K (2017) Therapeutic reasoning: planning, implementing, and evaluating the outcomes of therapy. In: RR Taylor ed. *Kielhofner's Model of Human Occupation: Theory and Application*. Philadelphia: Wolters Kluwer. 159–172.

Hagedorn R (2000) *Tools for Practice in Occupational Therapy.* Edinburgh: Churchill Livingstone.

Jamieson L, Parkinson S (2017) Unlocking potential: case formulation and measurable goals in a prison setting. *Occupational Therapy News, 25(3),* 36–38.

Korjonen H, Hughes E, Ford J, Keswani A (2016) *The Role of Case Studies as Evidence in Public Health.* London: UK Health Forum.

Kuyken W (2006) Evidence-based case formulation: is the emperor clothed? In: N Tarrier ed. *Case Formulation in Cognitive Behaviour Therapy: The Treatment of Challenging and Complex Cases.* Hove, Sussex: Routledge. 12–35.

Macneil CA, Hasty MK, Conus P, Berk M (2012) Is diagnosis enough to guide interventions in mental health? Using case formulation in clinical practice. *BMC Medicine 10*:111 DOI: 10.1186/1741-7015-10-111. Accessed 08/08/2019.

Page AC, Stritzke WGK, McLean NJ (2008) Toward science-informed supervision of clinical case formulation: a training model and supervision method. *Australian Psychologist, 43(2),* 88–95.

Parkinson S, Chester A, Cratchley S, Rowbottom J (2008) Application of the Model of Human Occupation Screening Tool (MOHOST assessment) in an acute psychiatric setting. *Occupational Therapy in Health Care, 22(2–3),* 63–75.

Parkinson S, Di Bona L, Fletcher N, Vecsey T, Wheeler K (2015) Profession-specific working in mental health: impacts for occupational therapists and service users. *New Zealand Journal of Occupational Therapy, 62(2),* 55–66.

Parkinson S, Lowe C, Keys K (2010) Professional development enhances the occupational therapy work environment. *British Journal of Occupational Therapy, 73(10),* 470–476.

Parkinson S, Shenfield M, Reece K, Elliott J (2011) Enhancing clinical reasoning through the use of evidence-based assessments, robust case formulations and measurable goals. *British Journal of Occupational Therapy 74(3),* 148–152.

Parkinson S, di Bona L, Fletcher N, Vecsey T, Wheeler K (2015) Profession-specific working in mental health: Impacts for occupational therapists and service users. *New Zealand Journal of Occupational Therapy, 62(2),* 55–66.

Pulido-Castelblanco D, Gómez MMN (2014) Clinical case formulation in a context of health. *Universitas Psychologica, 13(1),* 187–205.

Rainforth M, Laurenson M (2014) A literature review of case formulation to inform mental health practice. *Journal of Psychiatric and Mental Health Nursing, 21(3),* 206–213.

Richmond G (2017) Promoting Self-Efficacy in managing major depression. In: C Long, J Cronin-Davis, D Cotterill eds. *Occupational therapy in Practice for Mental Health.* Chichester: John Wiley and Sons 165–190.

Statewide Behaviour Intervention Service [SBIS] (2017) *Clinical Formulation Practice Guide: A Collaborative Approach.* Parramatta, Australia: Clinical Innovation and Governance, Ageing, Disability and Home Care, Department of Family and Community Services.

Taylor RR (2008) *The Intentional Relationship: Occupational Therapy and Therapeutic Use of Self.* Philadelphia: FA Davis.

Taylor RR ed. (2017) *Kielhofner's Model of Human Occupation.* 5th ed. Philadelphia: Wolters Kluwer.

Thompson BF (2012) Abductive reasoning and case formulation in complex cases. In: L Robertson ed. *Clinical Reasoning in Occupational Therapy.* Pondicherry: Wiley-Blackwell. 15–30.

Weiste E (2016) Formulations in occupational therapy: managing talk about psychiatric outpatients' emotional states. *Journal of Pragmatics, 105,* 59–73.

Whitton C, Small M, Lyon H, Barker L, Akiboh M (2016) The impact of case formulation meetings for teams, *Advances in Mental Health and Intellectual Disabilities, 10(2),* 145–157.

4   How are formulations compiled?

When considering how to compile a formulation, much has already been covered in previous chapters. In particular, the points made regarding the process of contextualisation are highly pertinent and worth repeating here.

The process of contextualisation involves comparing and contrasting a range of factors so that:

- limitations are viewed in the context of a person's strengths (Macneil et al. 2012, Thompson 2012, Brooks and Parkinson 2018)
- the person is viewed in the context of their environment (Statewide Behaviour Intervention Service [SBIS] 2017) including their socio-cultural environment (British Psychological Society [BPS] 2011)
- the person's subjective experience is viewed in the context of their observed performance (Brooks and Parkinson 2017)
- current performance is viewed in the context of personal history, including previous traumas (BPS 2011) or changes to personal circumstances (Lee and Kielhofner [posthumous] 2017)
- presenting issues are viewed in the context of clinical knowledge and theory (SBIS 2017)

However, a formulation does not simply list the above factors. Causal factors must be integrated and given that formulations focus primarily on personal meaning, the person's own story becomes an important integrative factor (BPS 2011). The integration of professional theories can also assist, and a cohesive formulation can be achieved through these two complementary techniques:

- integration into a narrative
- integration into a model

Integration into a narrative

Vertue and Haig (2008) describe case formulation as 'a complex narrative' (p1047) and it is certainly true that a formulation provides a way to manage complex information, but the narrative itself must be elegant and simple. A narrative is an account with a beginning, a middle, and an end (Greenhalgh 2016); and a formulation is similar in that it should have an unmistakeable directional flow. It offers a clear way of understanding simple questions such as 'Why is this person presenting in this way at this

DOI: 10.4324/9781003046301-4

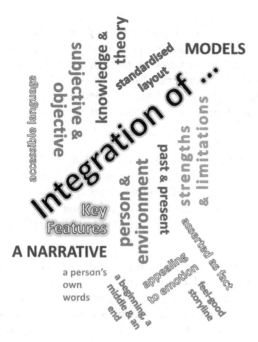

subjective & objective

knowledge & theory

accessible language

standardised layout

MODELS

Integration of ...

past & present

strengths & limitations

person & environment

Key Features

asserted as fact

A NARRATIVE

a person's own words

a beginning, a middle & an end

appealing to emotion

feel-good storyline

Figure 4.1 Key features of a formulation.

time and what is maintaining the situation?' (Robertson 2012) or, more simply, 'Why this person? why this problem? and why now?' (Macneil et al. 2012). The construction of a narrative, or storyline, makes it easier to grasp the multiple factors involved.

Before developing a narrative, one must first know one's audience and endeavour to make sure that the story will be comprehensible to everyone in this audience (Henderson and Martin 2014). This is likely to include the individual concerned as well as other non-professionals and workers from a range of other professions. The formulation should therefore be clear, organised (*ibid*), and presented in accessible language (BPS 2011), and must communicate something that is meaningful to the audience (Ryan 2007).

The message being communicated will become a narrative if it sets the scene and provides a coherent account of the characters and their motivations (Braddock and Dillard 2016). These characters will experience significant changes due to unforeseen events beyond their control, which may nevertheless be resolved through purposeful action (Ryan 2007). Given such a definition, the use of narrative is ideally suited for formulation. Furthermore, the sequence of narrative events should be causally linked and revolve around an event or events that are asserted as being fact (Ryan 2007). How, then, could any style of communication offer a more fitting shape for a case formulation?

Box 4.1   Author's note

by Sue Parkinson

Whenever I think about the importance of narrative, I am reminded of the words of Terry Pratchett – a favourite author of my husband's – and his ideas regarding the evolution and development of the human mind in the Science of the Discworld books. There is a fabulous explanation of why we are being optimistic when we refer to ourselves '*Homo sapiens*, meaning "wise man" in an appropriately dead language' (Pratchett et al. 2013, p4). This is not purely because men, or women, rarely seem to demonstrate the wisdom which we are credited with. It is because the thing that distinguishes us from other apes is our story-telling abilities. We should therefore be called *Pan narrans* – the storytelling ape (*ibid*), because,

> '*Our minds make stories, and stories make our minds. Each culture's Make-a-Human kit is built from stories, and maintained by stories. A story can be a rule for living according to one's culture, a useful survival trick … or a mental hypothesis about what might happen if we pursue a particular course*'
> (Pratchett et al. 2002, p327)

Although story-telling may have a negative reputation in the field of science, its use in case formulation is not without an evidence base. It is particularly relevant when communicating with non-expert audiences because it is naturally persuasive in nature, seeking as it does to capture interest and increase engagement (Dahlstrom 2014). Formulations strive to motivate all those involved, and there is a growing acceptance that a comprehensive story can affect the beliefs and actions of listeners and provide a powerful vehicle for changing opinion (Braddock and Dillard 2016). Individual facts may be singled out, disputed, resisted, or taken out of context, but the storyline mitigates against this (Moyer-Gusé 2008) by bringing disparate factors together into a single whole that holds the listeners' attention and can easily be remembered (Pipher 2006).

Trisha Greenhalgh (2016) makes a convincing argument for narrative being an essential tool for reports in the health sector. She cites the work of the renowned psychologist Jerome Bruner who divided human cognition into two forms: the logico-scientific mode which pays attention to empirical laws and the narrative mode which attempts to make sense, meaning, and purpose out of these scientific facts in relation to human experience. She acknowledges that,

> '*Even when based on real events, no story is an objective version of the truth (although importantly, the same might be said of a set of numbers or survey responses). Stories are subjective in that they convey one person's (or sometimes, a collective) version of events using a particular choice of words, metaphors, and styles. Stories are also intersubjective (i.e. they connect to, and respond to, the subjectivities of their reader(s) and listener(s) and are embodied in institutional and social practices. One person's story, told twice, is never the same. Different people tell different stories about the same event*' (p3)

According to Greenhalgh (2016), stories do not replicate empirical facts or appeal to logic. Instead, they appeal directly to our emotions by holding up a mirror to real life and reflecting something the listener or reader can recognise. She describes how this can be achieved through the use of certain literary devices: adhering to a given genre (e.g., tragedy or comedy), using metaphors effectively, ensuring the aesthetic appeal of the story, and upholding a moral order with good overcoming evil. In this way, case formulations might succeed by

- adopting a feel-good genre with a positive spin
- using the person's own metaphors to describe their view of life
- representing the person as the star of their own story
- indicating how the person can triumph in the end

If a narrative format seems ideally suited for formulations in general, then the fit could not be more perfect for occupational formulations. In 1991, Mattingly asserted that narrative reasoning is a central mode of clinical reasoning in occupational therapy. Narrative reasoning supports an occupational therapist to move from objective observation to an appreciation of the person's subjective experience, and is characterised by a focus on the individual when attempting to understand a person's experiences (Schell and Schell 2008). This focus is necessarily located within the person's life story because people's identities are understood in the context of ongoing life events which would appear arbitrary and meaningless without something to connect them together (Christiansen 1999). A life story provides coherence and unity which affords a degree of consistency to the actions of each individual; so in constructing stories we create a framework to fashion identities in a way that makes sense to the person and to those whose stories interconnect with that person (*ibid*).

Narrative reasoning may even culminate in the creation of a collaborative story (Schell and Schell 2008). In recent years, however, occupational therapists appear to have been more interested in how narrative might be used as an assessment medium or a medium for specific interventions, rather than the stage between assessment and intervention. For instance, occupational therapists have described the importance of narrative interviewing (Mattingly and Lawler 2000) and the value of a history-based interview (Ennals and Fossey 2009). They have also promoted narrative storytelling as intervention for people recovering from trauma (Moore 2017) and digital storytelling as an intervention to enhance the reflection of occupational therapy students (Skarpass and Jamissen 2016). Likewise, psychologists and psychotherapists have also noted the potential of 'narrative therapy' (Dallos and Stedman 2014) including the therapeutic merit of summarising new stories learned in therapy sessions in a series of letters (Harper and Spellman 2014).

Despite few references to occupational formulation *per se*, the case for narrative occupational formulation has been growing steadily, especially in the minds of occupational therapists fortunate enough to have worked with or be influenced by Gary Kielhofner, who originally created the Model of Human Occupation (MOHO) along with Janice Burke (Kielhofner and Burke 1980).

- in 1993, Platts viewed MOHO as essential for *formulating* occupational therapy treatment plans
- in 1999, Mentrup, Niehaus, and Kielhofner presented their ideas for using MOHO as a guide to formulating and implementing therapy
- in 2001, Braveman and Helfrich highlighted the unifying properties of '*self-stories*' and the use of '*narrative analysis*' for making sense of people's occupational lives
- in 2002, Auzmendia and others contributed to Kielhofner's third edition of his seminal textbook – 'Model of Human Occupation: theory and application' – by producing a chapter entitled '*Re-crafting occupational narratives*'

- in 2004, Goldstein, Kielhofner and Paul-Ward emphasised the crucial role that *occupational narratives* have in situating where people see themselves in 'a plot that integrates past, present, and future', and stated that narratives could help to predict a person's response to occupational therapy
- in 2008, Kielhofner and Forsyth proposed that therapeutic reasoning progresses from gathering information (assessment) to '*creating a conceptualisation of the client that includes strengths and weaknesses*' (p149)
- in the same year, Keponen and Launiainen wrote about using MOHO to nurture an occupational focus in occupational therapists' professional reasoning, including applying MOHO concepts and assessment information into a *formulation*
- in 2009, Ikiugu, Smallfield, and Condit suggested that, although occupational therapists might use multiple models, MOHO might be viewed as the most suitable 'organising model of practice' when producing a *collaborative formulation*
- finally, in 2017, the term '*occupational formulation*' is used by Forsyth in the fifth edition of 'Kielhofner's Model of Human Occupation' (ed. Taylor). In this same book, Melton and her colleagues demonstrated how occupational *narratives* evolve over time and how MOHO can be used to explain the process

Integration into a model

Occupational therapy is not the only profession to utilise models in case formulation. The Good Practice Guidelines on the use of psychological formulation (BPS 2011) recommends that formulations are 'informed by a range of models' and that these models are integrated rather than simply being listed (p29). Drawing on these models will assist the fulfilment of other criteria, in that psychological formulations should be grounded in psychological theory and evidence and make theoretical sense (*ibid*). It follows, therefore, that occupational formulations will draw upon occupational models and make use of the best theories and research available.

Box 4.2   Author's note

by Dr Rob Brooks

When I worked as a clinician, I often used to summarise the issues facing a person using subheadings for the key occupational domains: self-care, productivity, and leisure. This was never entirely satisfactory as the domains often interlink and the issues facing one person might be largely within the sphere of self-care, while the issues facing another might be mostly relating to productivity. I also experimented with presenting information using MOHO concepts and I continue to encounter this structure being used by practising clinicians. The difficulty is that concepts like volition, habituation, performance, and the environment are technical terms with particular connotations that may not be understood by our audiences. More than this, volition, habituation, performance, and the environment are dynamically interrelated and are equally important, so they do not provide a narrative flow.

Rather than trying to educate the general population in using our professional language, or expecting our colleagues to grasp the nuances of occupational therapy practice, it would be better if we wrote in a style that is accessible to all. The second section of this book describes how to construct an occupational formulation using a flowing narrative style (Brooks and Parkinson 2018) with a beginning, a middle, and an end (Jamieson and Parkinson 2017). Volition, habituation, performance capacity, and the environment will still have their part to play, but they are not centre stage. Instead, therapists use other MOHO terms to demonstrate that they understand a person's occupational *identity* or where the person has come from; they provide an objective account of the person's occupational *competence* or where they are now; and they negotiate the issues affecting occupational *adaptation* that will provide direction for the person as they navigate the way forward.

Models can be integrated into report formats and can also form the basis of a consistent layout for a formulation. Indeed, 'manualised approaches' are recommended in Cognitive Behavioural Therapy guidelines (Kuyken 2006) as a means of standardising practice and maintaining standards. Likewise, Behavioural Activation formulations tend to follow a set format, starting with antecedent behaviours (Richmond 2017), while Macneil et al. (2012) recommend following the 5Ps model in mental health practice:

- Presenting problem
- Predisposing factors
- Precipitating factors
- Perpetuating factors
- Protective/positive factors

Within occupational therapy, it has been argued that models are essential to contemporary practice and provide occupational therapists with an organisational structure for communicating and documenting complex processes (Joosten 2015). A range of models exist and could be used to inform occupational formulations, but Loftus and Higgs (2008) recommend that ideas about service users are constructed within a single conceptual framework. In this instance, the Model of Human Occupation (MOHO) (ed. Taylor 2017) will be referred to throughout the remainder of the book (see Figure 4.2). Not only are there clear indications that it is one of the most widely taught·conceptual models of practice in of occupational therapy (Ashby and Chandler 2010), but it also seems to be the most researched (Vessby and Kjellberg 2010) and the most used in occupational therapy practice (Lee et al. 2008). Moreover, its particular suitability for guiding the collaborative formulation of therapeutic goals is recognised even by those who recommend combining multiple models (Ikiugu et al. 2009). However, readers may choose to integrate other occupational models of practice into their occupational formulations.

MOHO's reputation for being an excellent model on which to base an occupational formulation owes a great deal to Kirsty Forsyth, who has co-authored multiple articles associating the model with formulation (Forsyth et al. 2005b, Harrison and Forsyth 2005, Wimpenny et al. 2006, Melton et al. 2008, Shinohara et al. 2012). To date, however, many of these articles state that formulations are created without fully explaining how they are constructed. Also, although Forsyth describes the role of

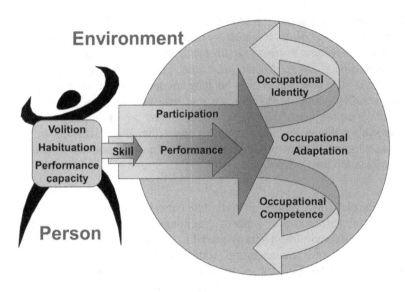

Figure 4.2 Model of Human Occupation.
      (*Source: image adapted from Kielhofner's MOHO textbook [ed. Taylor 2017]*).

occupational formulation in the 2017 edition of the MOHO textbook, and offers a comprehensive list of reflective questions that will assist in building a formulation, as well as sharing an example summary, the full structure of a formulation is not described.

MOHO fits well with occupational formulation, partly because it offers a wide range of assessments that support occupation and person-centred, evidence-based practice. These assist the therapist to answer key occupational questions relating to the model's main concepts (Cubie and Kaplan 1982), including volition, habituation, performance (including performance capacity, performance skills, performance of activities and participation in occupation), and the environment (see Table 4.1).

Table 4.1 Example questions based on the Model of Human Occupation (Parkinson 2014)

- Does the person expect to be able to do [an occupation]? (personal causation)
- Does the person enjoy [an occupation]? (interests)
- How important is [an occupation] to the person? (values)
- Do the person's responsibilities support or interfere with their ability to participate in [an occupation]? (roles)
- Is [an occupation] integrated into the person's routines? (habits)
- Does any impairment affect the person's ability to participate in [an occupation]? (performance capacity)
- Does the person have adequate motor, process and communication & interaction skills to perform [an occupation]? (skills)
- Where can the person participate in [an occupation]? (physical space)
- Are there sufficient resources for the person to participate in [an occupation]? (physical objects)
- Who could support the person to participate in [an occupation]? (social environment)

More than this, the model explains how the above concepts are necessary for occupational adaptation – our ability to make needed changes so that we can continue to engage in chosen activities and occupations, or develop new occupations (O'Brien and Kielhofner [posthumous] 2017). Occupational adaptation is viewed as the highest achievement and depends on a person developing a secure sense of their occupational identity along with the occupational competence to maintain that identity.

Box 4.3   Author's note

by Dr Rob Brooks

In our 2018 opinion piece, Sue and I presented a universal structure for occupational formulation consisting of Occupational Influences, Occupational Presentation, and Occupational Focus. This three-part structure describes the past, the present, and a possible future regarding a person's occupational life. I believe that this universal structure can be used to underpin and integrate the constructs from most of the occupational models we use in practice. I would also suggest that it enables us to apply what we have learnt from occupational science in relation a person's experience of occupational justice – for example, alienation, deprivation, marginalisation, imbalance, and apartheid.

Table 4.2 presents the Universal Occupational Formulation Structure, which illustrates how it is mapped to a narrative structure. Table 4.2 also provides an example of a MOHO-based formulation structure using the constructs of occupational identity, competence, and adaptation. This, too, is mapped to an overall narrative structure.

We will be using this MOHO-based structure for the rest of this book to illustrate how to write occupational formulations and goals. Each formulation sets out to compare and contrast a person's identity and competence, with all information feeding into these two items. So instead of listing all that is known about a person's volition, habituation, performance capacity, and environment (and the myriad components within these four main concepts), a MOHO-based formulation is able to provide the much sought-after simplicity by encapsulating the therapist's perspective in two neatly matched halves. Moreover, whereas the full meaning of the terms volition, habituation, performance capacity, and environment are not well-understood by non-occupational therapists, the terms identity and competence are technical enough to bolster professional credibility and still have currency in common parlance.

Crucially, the concepts of occupational identity and occupational competence create a natural flow or storyline within the formulation. There is a clear hierarchy in which the person's identity is given primary importance, and this needs to be understood first, because competence in MOHO is defined as how well a person is able to maintain this identity. The narrative flow also has a clear direction because occupational identity is developed over time, starting with a person's early experiences, and occupational competence is most apparent in a person's current presentation and circumstances.

Table 4.2 Three interlinking structures for an occupational formulation

A narrative structure	A universal structure	A MOHO-based structure
A beginning, The past – where the person has come from	Occupational influences	Occupational identity
A middle, The present – where the person is now	Occupational presentation	Occupational competence
An end, The future – the future direction of therapy	Occupational focus	Key issues for occupational adaptation

- A narrative structure (Jamieson and Parkinson 2017).
- A universal structure (Brooks and Parkinson 2018).
- A MOHO-based structure (Parkinson et al. 2011, Forsyth 2017, Brooks and Parkinson 2018).

References

Ashby J, Chandler B (2010) An exploratory study of the occupation-focused models included in occupational therapy professional education programmes. *British Journal of Occupational Therapy*, *73(12)*, 616–624.

Auzmendia AL, de las Heras CG, Kielhofner G, Miranda C (2002). Recrafting occupational narratives. In: G Kielhofner ed. *Model of Human Occupation: Theory and Application*. 4th ed. Baltimore: Lippincott Williams & Wilkins. 359–380.

Braddock K, Dillard JP (2016) Meta-analytic evidence for the persuasive effect of narratives on beliefs, attitudes, intentions, and behaviors. *Communication Monographs*, *83(4)*, 446–467.

Braveman B, Helfrich CA (2001) Occupational identity: exploring the narratives of three men living with AIDS. *Journal of Occupational Science*, *8(2)*, 25–31.

British Psychological Society [BPS] (2011) *Good Practice Guidelines on the Use of Psychological Formulation*. Leicester: BPS.

Brooks R, Parkinson S (2018) Occupational formulation: a three-part structure. *British Journal of Occupational Therapy*, *81(3)*, 177–179.

Christiansen CH (1999) Defining lives: occupation as identity: an essay on competence, coherence and the creation of meaning. *American Journal of Occupational Therapy*, *53(6)*, 547–558.

Cubie SH, Kaplan K (1982) A case analysis method for the Model of Human Occupation. *American Journal of Occupational Therapy*, *36(10)*, 645–656.

Dahlstrom MF (2014) Using narratives and storytelling to communicate science with nonexpert audiences. *Proceedings of the National Academy of Sciences of the United States of America 16*(111 Suppl 4), 13614–13620. doi: 10.1073/pnas.1320645111.

Dallos R and Stedman J (2014) Integrative formulation in practice: a dynamic multi-level approach. In: Johnstone L, Dallos R eds. *Formulation in Psychology and Psychotherapy: Make Sense of People's Problems*. 2nd ed. Hove, Sussex: Routledge. 191–216.

Ennals P, Fossey E (2009) Using the OPHI-II to support people with mental illness in their recovery. *Occupational Therapy in Mental Health*, *25(2)*, 138–150.

Forsyth K (2017) Therapeutic reasoning: planning, implementing, and evaluating the outcomes of therapy. In: RR Taylor ed. *Kielhofner's Model of Human Occupation: Theory and Application*. Philadelphia: Wolters Kluwer. 159–172.

Forsyth K, Duncan EAS, Mann LS (2005b) Scholarship of Practice in the United Kingdom: an occupational therapy service case study. *Occupational Therapy in Health Care, 19(1–2)*, 17–29.

Goldstein, K, Kielhofner G, and Paul-Ward A (2004) Occupational narratives and the therapeutic process. *Australian Occupational Therapy Journal, 51(3)*, 119–124.

Greenhalgh T (2016) *Cultural Contexts of Health: The Use of Narrative Research in the Health Sector* (Health Evidence Network Synthesis Report 49). Copenhagen: World Health Organisation.

Harper D and Spellman D (2014) Formulation and narrative therapy. In: L Johnstone L, R Dallos eds. *Formulation in Psychology and Psychotherapy: Make Sense of People's Problems.* 2nd ed. Hove, Sussex: Routledge. 96–120.

Harrison M, Forsyth K (2005) Developing a vision for therapists working within child and adolescent mental health services: poised or paused for action? *British Journal of Occupational Therapy, 68(4)*, 181–185.

Henderson SW, Andrés Martin (2014) Case formulation and integration of information in child and adolescent mental health. In: JM Rey ed. *IACAPAP e-Textbook of Child and Adolescent Mental Health.* Geneva: International Association for Child and Adolescent Psychiatry and Allied Professions.

Ikiugu MN, Smallfield S, Condit C (2009) A framework for combining theoretical conceptual practice models in occupational therapy practice. *Canadian Journal of Occupational Therapy, 76(3)*, 162–170.

Jamieson L, Parkinson S (2017) Unlocking potential: case formulation and measurable goals in a prison setting. *Occupational Therapy News, 25(3)*, 36–38.

Joosten AV (2015) Contemporary occupational therapy: our occupational therapy models are essential to occupation centred practice. *Australian Occupational Therapy Journal, 62(3)*, 219–222. DOI: 10.1111/1440-1630.12186.

Kielhofner G, Burke JP (1980) A Model of Human Occupation, Part 1. Conceptual framework and content. *American Journal of Occupational Therapy, 34(9)*, 572–581.

Kielhofner G, Forsyth K (2008) Occupational engagement: how clients achieve change. In: G Kielhofner ed. *Model of Human Occupation: Theory and Application.* 4th ed. Baltimore: Lippincott, Williams & Wilkins, 101–109.

Kuyken W (2006) Evidence-based case formulation: is the emperor clothed? In: N Tarrier ed. *Case formulation in Cognitive Behaviour Therapy: The Treatment of Challenging and Complex Cases.* Hove, Sussex: Routledge. 12–35.

Lee SW, Kielhofner G [posthumous] (2017) Habituation: patterns of daily occupation. In: RR Taylor ed. *Kielhofner's Model of Human Occupation: Theory and Application.* Philadelphia: Wolters Kluwer. 57–73.

Lee SW, Taylor R, Kielhofner G, Fisher G (2008) Theory use in practice: a national survey of therapists who use the Model of Human Occupation. *American Journal of Occupational Therapy, 62(1)*, 106–117.

Loftus S, Higgs J (2008) Learning the language of clinical reasoning. In: J Higgs, MA Jones, S Loftus, N Christensen eds. *Clinical Reasoning in the Health Professions.* 3rd ed. Oxford: Butterworth-Heinemann, 399–448.

Macneil CA, Hasty MK, Conus P, Berk M (2012) Is diagnosis enough to guide interventions in mental health? Using case formulation in clinical practice. *BMC Medicine 10*:111 DOI: 10. 1186/1741-7015-10-111. Accessed 08/08/2019.

Mattingly C (1991) The narrative nature of clinical reasoning. *American Journal of Occupational Therapy, 45(11)*, 998–1005.

Mattingly C, Lawler M (2000) Learning from stories: narrative interviewing in cross-cultural research. *Scandinavian Journal of Occupational Therapy, 7(1)*, 4–14.

Melton J, Forsyth K, Metherall A, Robinson J, Hill J, Quick L (2008). Program redesign based on the model of human occupation: inpatient services for people experiencing acute mental illness in the UK. *Occupational Therapy in Health-Care, 22(2–3)*, 37–50.

Melton J, Holzmueller RP, Keponen R, Nygard L, Munger K, Kielhofner G [posthumous] (2017) Crafting occupational life. In: RR Taylor ed. *Kielhofner's Model of Human Occupation: Theory and Application*. Philadelphia: Lippincott, Williams and Wilkins. 123–139.

Mentrup C, Niehaus A, Kielhofner G (1999) Applying the model of human occupation in work-focused rehabilitation: a case illustration. *Work, 12(1)*, 61–70.

Moore T, 2017, Strengths-based narrative storytelling as therapeutic intervention for refugees in Greece. *WFOT Bulletin, 73(1)*, 45–51.

Moyer-Gusé E (2008) Toward a theory of entertainment persuasion: explaining the persuasive effects of entertainment-education messages. *Communication Theory, 18(3)*, 407–425. doi:10.1111/j.1468-2885.2008.00328.x.

O'Brien JC, Kielhofner G [posthumous] (2017) The interaction between the person and the environment. In: RR Taylor ed., *Kielhofner's Model of Human Occupation*. 5th ed. Philadelphia: Wolters Kluwer. 24–37.

Parkinson S (2014) *Recovery Through Activity: Increasing Participation in Everyday Life*. London: Speechmark Publishing.

Parkinson S, Shenfield M, Reece K, Elliott J (2011) Enhancing clinical reasoning through the use of evidence-based assessments, robust case formulations and measurable goals. *British Journal of Occupational Therapy 74(3)*, 148–152.

Pipher M (2006) *Writing to Change the World*. New York: Riverhead Books.

Platts L (1993) Social Role Valorisation and the Model of Human Occupation: a comparative analysis for work with people with a learning disability in the community. *British Journal of Occupational Therapy, 56(8)*, 278–282.

Pratchett, T, Stewart I, Cohen J (2002) *The Science of the Discworld II: The Globe*. London: Ebury Press.

Pratchett, T, Stewart I, Cohen J (2013) *The Science of the Discworld IV: Judgement Day*. London: Ebury Press

Richmond Gill (2017) Promoting self-efficacy in managing major depression, chapter 8. In: Long C Cronin-Davis J Cotterill D , eds., *Occupational Therapy in Practice for Mental Health*. John Wiley and Sons. 165–190.

Robertson L (2012) *Clinical Reasoning in Occupational Therapy: Controversies in Practice*. Chichester: John Wiley and Sons.

Ryan M (2007) Toward a definition of narrative. In: D Herman ed. *The Cambridge Companion to Narrative*. New York, NY: Cambridge University Press. 22–35.

Schell BA, Schell JW (2008) *Clinical and Professional Reasoning in Occupational Therapy*. Philadelphia: Lippincott Williams & Wilkins.

Shinohara K, Yamada T, Kobayashi N, Forsyth K (2012) The Model of Human Occupation-based intervention for patients with stroke: a randomised trial. *Hong Kong Journal of Occupational Therapy, 22(2)*, 60–69.

Skarpass LS, Jamissen G (2016) Digital storytelling as poetic reflection in Occupational Therapy education: an empirical study. *The Open Journal of Occupational Therapy, 4(3)*, Article 5. Accessed 08/08/2019.

Statewide Behaviour Intervention Service [SBIS] (2017) *Clinical Formulation Practice Guide: A Collaborative Approach*. Parramatta, Australia: Clinical Innovation and Governance, Ageing, Disability and Home Care, Department of Family and Community Services.

Taylor RR ed. (2017) *Kielhofner's Model of Human Occupation*. 5th ed. Philadelphia: Wolters Kluwer.

Thompson BF (2012) Abductive reasoning and case formulation in complex cases. In: L Robertson ed. *Clinical Reasoning in Occupational Therapy*. Pondicherry: Wiley-Blackwell. 15–30.

Vertue FM, Haig BD (2008) An abductive perspective on clinical reasoning and case formulation. *Journal of Clinical Psychology*, *64*(*9*), 1046–1068.

Vessby K, Kjellberg A (2010) Participation in occupational therapy research: a literature review. *British Journal of Occupational Therapy*, *73*(*7*), 319–326.

Wimpenny K, Forsyth K, Jones C, Evans E, Colley J (2006) Group reflective supervision: thinking with theory to develop practice. *British Journal of Occupational Therapy*, *69*(*9*), 423–428.

Part II

Constructing occupational formulations and goals

5 Structuring the Occupational Identity section

A key component of the therapeutic process

Our occupational identities are integral to our sense of who we are and reflect the whole of our occupational lives and everything in which we participate. Simply put, occupational identity,

> '... implies that people are what they do. People engage in those activities for which they find meaning or pleasure. They repeat patterns of behaviour that fulfil them and serve to create an identity or sense of purpose'
>
> (O'Brien and Kielhofner [posthumous] 2017, p33)

Accordingly, occupational therapists must take note of a person's occupational identity at each stage of the therapeutic process.

- in the *assessment* phase, it is recommended that therapists explore the occupations that are most meaningful to an individual as this can provide a way to understanding their unique identity (Unruh 2004)
- the resulting *formulation* articulates the person's identity and conforms to Christiansen's belief that identity depicts 'a central figure in a self-narrative or life story that provides coherence and meaning for everyday events and life itself' (Christiansen 1999, p550)
- when *planning* interventions, it should be recognised that motivation depends on having a sense of identity (Christiansen 1999). An individual's acknowledged identity can, therefore, provide a framework or a platform for setting therapeutic goals (*ibid*) and may even be essential for collaborative goal-setting (Unruh 2004)
- *interventions* aim to offer new opportunities for people to express themselves in order to rebuild lost identities or create new identities (Christiansen 1999) and begin the process of reconstructing their lives
- the *review* stage could be said to be supporting individuals to link their past and future occupational identities (Vrkljan and Polgar 2007)

Highlighting participation in occupational roles

Our sense of identity is routinely bound by what we do – our occupations and the roles they are connected with. In social conversation, when we are getting to know others, we automatically enquire what they do (Unruh 2004). Similarly, when we happen

DOI: 10.4324/9781003046301-5

upon strangers and ask who they are, they may legitimise their presence by naming their role, and in this way, occupations are commonly used to communicate a sense of identity (Phelan and Kinsella 2009).

Whether our occupations are related to self-care, leisure, or productivity (work-related activities), they seem to contribute to how we perceive ourselves, our social relationships, and our sense of belonging in the world (Blank et al. 2015). Unsurprisingly, therefore, participation in occupation is deemed to be a central determinant in developing identity (Christiansen 1999). It is believed that having a key role gives us a sense of belonging and of being included in the world (Blank et al. 2015), thereby affecting well-being and life-satisfaction (Christiansen 1999).

Identities are generated and modified over the course of time and space. Thus, comprehending a person's occupational identity necessarily involves an appreciation of their history of occupational participation (Kielhofner 2008) as well as their varied social environments (Christiansen 1999). In fact, a single person may have multiple identities that contribute to their sense of self and these have the potential to encompass global, local, and personal interactions across the person's lifespan, including:

- the person's place in the social, cultural, and political dimensions of the wider world (Phelan and Kinsella 2009)
- the person's public identities and private identities (Unruh 2004) including their work role and the social value or status attached to this (Blank et al. 2015), as well as their solo participation in meaningful interests (Phelan and Kinsella 2009)

Box 5.1   Author's note

by Dr Rob Brooks

When capturing a person's identity in an occupational formulation, it makes sense to consider the roles the person has had in the past as well as the roles they have in the present, and the roles that they are seeking in the future (without assuming that someone wants to return to past occupations). In this way, the narrative is rooted in the past but has a natural flow as the timeline moves forward. It is also a good idea to provide key details regarding the person's roles. For instance:

- If they have been a worker, what jobs have they had?
- If they are a student, which subjects are they studying?
- If they are part of a family, who are their family members?
- If they participate in a hobby, what does it involve?

Their roles might be formal with clear responsibilities or more informal with characteristics that the person takes upon themselves, such as playing the joker, or being the strong and silent type, the critic, or the socialiser. The objective is to capture how the person sees themselves, so you should use the person's own words as much as possible.

Emphasising personal meaning

Ultimately, a person's composite identity rests on the person's own interpretation of their participation in the context of their relationships with others (Christiansen 1999). The person's own view of their identity is crucial, and therapists must seek to grasp the meaning that individuals place on their experiences at an affective, cognitive, and spiritual level (Unruh 2004, Phelan and Kinsella 2009). They also need to recognise the inevitable changes to an individual's participation in meaningful occupations that have been made in response to life turning points and significant events (Vrkljan and Polgar 2007).

Just as changes to occupational participation can injure a person's occupational identity, changes can also provide the means for healing. Those with the capacity for self-determination learn that identity can be crafted and become a blueprint for future action (O'Brien and Kielhofner [posthumous] 2017). This realisation prompts many people to seek occupational participation quite spontaneously as a means for influencing identity change. Their object may be to distance themselves from unwanted or spoiled identities or to cope with those that have been threatened, to create a brand new identity or to reconnect with a previous valued identity, and eventually to integrate separate identities to form a coherent whole (Blank et al. 2015).

Box 5.2 Author's note

by Dr Rob Brooks

I recommend that you refrain from using the person's own words if there is any risk of reinforcing catastrophic feelings. For instance, the person might say that they 'hate' someone but would accept the less inflammatory statement that they 'have a difficult relationship' with them. This does not ignore the person's viewpoint – it is simply a case of reframing their feelings to allow for more hopeful outcomes. For the same reason, as well as recording any difficult or traumatic feelings, I always make a note of any positive feelings. In this way, a person's identity is depicted with light and shade rather than being overwhelmingly bleak, and I demonstrate my belief in the person's strengths and their potential to change.

Identity and the Model of Human Occupation

The relationship between occupation and identity has been clearly articulated by the Model of Human Occupation (MOHO) (ed. Taylor 2017). Since the model was first developed in 1980, it has emphasised the importance of 'volition' (comprising thoughts and feelings) and 'habituation' (including roles and habits). Some of these concepts are also found in Christiansen's celebrated 1999 Eleanor Clarke Slagle Lecture, *Defining lives: occupation as identity*, in which values, desires, and goals are associated with the notion of identity, as well as roles and relationships. As might be expected, his work is referred to when the term 'occupational identity' is defined in the Model of Human Occupation (Kielhofner 2008, de las Heras de Pablo et al. 2017a) (see Figure 5.1).

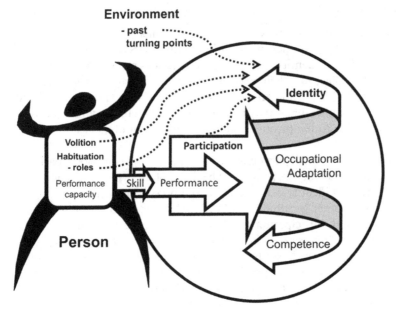

Figure 5.1 MOHO concepts that contribute to a sense of identity.
(*Source: image adapted from Kielhofner's MOHO textbook* [ed.Taylor 2017]).

Box 5.3   Author's note

by Sue Parkinson

According to MOHO, occupational identity is formed by participation in past and present roles, relationships, interests, and life turning points, and is set in a volitional context that reflects a person's satisfaction, personal causation, and goals. These terms provide a form of shorthand and help to structure professional reasoning for occupational therapists, but I would not expect non-occupational therapists to share the same level of understanding. I believe that the section heading – Occupational Identity – is sufficient to communicate a professional stance on its own without being baffling to the layperson. After that, although the section may be steeped in MOHO concepts to the trained eye, MOHO language does not need to take centre stage (see Table 5.1).

Table 5.1 Basic content of an occupational identity section

1. Past & present roles and relationships + Volition[*]
2. Life turning points + Volition[*]
3. Past & present interests + Volition[*]

Note
[*] Volition = feelings related to values, satisfaction, appraisal of ability, expectation of success & goals.

The Model of Human Occupation (MOHO) describes occupational identity as *'a composite sense of who one is and wishes to become as an occupational being generated from one's history of occupational participation. One's volition, habituation, and experience as a lived body are all integrated into occupational identity'* (Kielhofner 2008, p106). Along with occupational competence, occupational identity is conceptualised as a direct consequence of occupational participation. It *'serves as a means of self-definition and as a blue-print for upcoming action'* (de las Heras de Pablo et al. 2017a, p117). It follows, therefore, that MOHO encourages occupational therapists to make every attempt to understand a person's occupational identity.

This task has been assisted by a variety of MOHO-based assessments including the Role Checklist – Version 3 (Scott and Haggerty 1984) and version 2.1 of the Occupational Performance History Interview (OPHI-II) (Kielhofner et al. 2004).

The Role Checklist (Scott, 2019) is available from MOHO Web (www.moho.uic. edu) and has recently been revised, allowing individuals to identify the key roles in their lives and to rate their satisfaction with these roles. Ten roles are included in the checklist:

- student
- worker
- volunteer
- caregiver
- home-maintainer
- friend
- family member
- religious participant
- hobbyist/amateur
- participant in an organisation

The Occupational Performance History Interview Version 2.1 (OPHI II) (Kielhofner et al. 2004) is available from MOHO Web (www.moho.uic.edu) and supports therapists to assess whether an individual

- has personal goals and projects
- identifies a desired occupational lifestyle
- expects success
- accepts responsibility
- appraises abilities and limitations
- has commitments and values
- recognises identity and obligations
- has interests
- has felt effective
- has found meaning and satisfaction in past lifestyle
- has made occupational choices

Although roles, relationships, and habits are implicit in a person's obligations, lifestyle, and choices, the main emphasis of the Identity section in the OPHI-II is clearly about volition. The close link between volition and occupational identity is reinforced

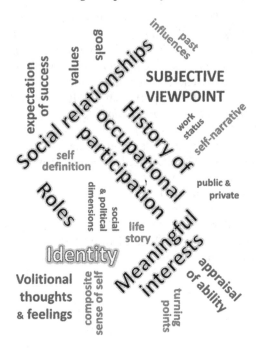

Figure 5.2 Occupational identity.

in Kielhofner's Model of Human Occupation latest textbook (ed. Taylor 2017) which states that occupational identity is constructed as the volitional process develops and changes (de las Heras de Pablo et al. 2017a). Furthermore, Occupational identity is described as an integrated composite of volitional components including personal causation, interests, roles identity, volitional anticipation, preferences, and choices (*ibid*).

- personal causation – a sense that you can cause things to happen based on your appraisal of your abilities and your expectation of success
- interests – pursuits that you find enjoyable and satisfying
- role identity – a sense of who you are with respect to your roles and relationships
- values – what is important to you and what you feel a sense of obligation towards
- volitional anticipation – your desired routines and environmental expectations
- preferences – your ideal way of life and preferred ways of doing things
- choices – your day-to-day decisions and future goals

Box 5.4   Author's note

by Sue Parkinson

In order to convey the meaning that a person attributes to their roles and the turning points in their lives, the identity section in an occupational formulation should be written from the person's subjective viewpoint. For this reason, I try to include the person's feelings in every single sentence by linking each aspect of their identity to their volition – their values or appraisal of ability, their expectation of success, satisfaction, choices, or goals (see Table 5.2).

Rather than using the sanitised language of a scientific report, I try to reflect the authentic feeling of the individual using plain language. This means that

- instead of writing that they 'appear to enjoy' something – a phrase that emphasises objectivity or the therapist's viewpoint – I might write about the things that they 'love'
- instead of writing that something is their 'goal', I am more likely to simply record that they 'want' to do something
- instead of writing that the person 'identifies' themselves with various roles, I would write that the roles are 'important' to them
- instead of referring to a person's 'sense of capacity' or 'sense of efficacy', I would describe how well the person 'feels' that they are able to do things, and describe their 'hope' for the future

Table 5.2 Top tips for the occupational identity section

- Give a sense of the whole person, showing that you understand where they are coming from
- Write this section and the competence section in user-friendly terms, avoiding the use of technical language
- Aim to tell the person's story – to give the person a voice
- Start by describing the person's occupational history – their childhood if relevant, as well as previous jobs and relationships
- Quote the person's own words, except when these might be regretted, for instance, when they may hurt others or make a situation appear worse than it is
- Avoid using phrases that may cast doubt on the person's viewpoint, such as 'apparently', 'he reports that, or 'she states that'
- Provide key details by naming significant jobs and particular interests
- Whenever a role or experience is mentioned, comment on how the person felt or feels about it
- Always include some positive feelings, including what the person is interested in and values, and what they hope for the future
- If the person cannot identify any positives, then wait until these are revealed by further assessment or by applying the Remotivation Process (de las Heras de Pablo et al. 2019) before attempting a formulation
- Start and end this section with positives
- Instead of starting a sentence with a positive followed by 'but', try inverting the information so that the sentence starts with 'Despite ...' and ends on a positive
- When referring to the person's life turning points, consider including their view of their illness, or their admission, or the offence they committed if they have been admitted to a secure service
- Emphasise the person's subjective viewpoint – what they feel, believe, think, like, enjoy, aspire to do, and find important
- N.B. save any objective descriptions of the person's routines, skills, performance, and their current environmental context for the competence section

References

Blank AA, Harries P, Reynolds F (2015) 'Without occupation you don't exist': occupational engagement and mental illness. *Journal of Occupational Science, 22(2)*, 197–209.

Christiansen CH (1999) Defining lives: occupation as identity: an essay on competence, coherence and the creation of meaning. *American Journal of Occupational Therapy, 53(6)*, 547–558.

de las Heras CG, Llerana V, Kielhofner G [posthumous] (2019) *The Remotivation Process: Progressive Intervention for Individuals With Severe Volitional Challenges: A User's Manual. Version 2.0*. Chicago: University of Illinois at Chicago.

de las Heras de Pablo, Fan C-W, Kielhofner G [posthumous] (2017a) Dimensions of Doing. In RR Taylor, ed. *Kielhofner's Model of Human Occupation: Ttheory and Application.* Philadelphia: Wolters Kluwer. 107–122.

Kielhofner G (2008) *Model of Human Occupation: Theory and Application*, 4th ed. Baltimore: Lippincott, Williams & Wilkins.

Kielhofner G, Mallinson T, Crawford C, Nowak M, Rigby M, Henry A, Walens D (2004) *Occupational Performance History Interview (OPHI-II), Version 2.1*. Chicago: University of Illinois.

O'Brien JC, Kielhofner G [posthumous] (2017) The interaction between the person and the environment. In: RR Taylor ed., *Kielhofner's Model of Human Occupation.* 5th ed. Philadelphia: Wolters Kluwer. 24–37.

Phelan S, Kinsella EA (2009) Occupational Identity: engaging socio-cultural perspectives. *Journal of Occupational Science, 16(2)*, 85–91.

Scott, PJ (2019) The Role Checklist v3. *Chicago:University of Illinois, 4(2)*, 39–58.

Taylor RR ed. (2017) *Kielhofner's Model of Human Occupation*. 5th ed. Philadelphia: Wolters Kluwer.

Unruh AM (2004) Reflections on: "So … What Do You Do?" Occupation and the construction of identity. *Canadian Journal of Occupational Therapy, 71(5)*, 290–295.

Vrkljan BH, Polgar JM (2007) Linking occupational participation and occupational identity: an exploratory study of the transition from driving to driving cessation in older adulthood. *Journal of Occupational Science, 14(1)*, 30–39.

6 Structuring the Occupational Competence section

A dynamic concept

It has been proposed that occupational therapy should communicate its importance 'simply, easily, and clearly' as 'the discipline concerned with enabling occupational competence' (Polatajko 1992, p189), and this abbreviated definition may well be sufficient for the general population. However, Polatajko's definition goes on to say that occupational competence is 'determined by the interaction of the individual and the environment' (p196) and furthermore that

> 'occupational competence is the product of the dynamic interaction between the environment and the individual, each changing in response to the other' (p197)

This dynamic interaction between the environment and the individual (or should one say the individual's identity?) is a complex process. One that merits further investigation or, without careful scrutiny, poses a risk that a person's occupational competence might not be captured fully.

The concept of a person's identity is known to be abstract, nebulous, and hard to pin down, whereas a person's competency is often thought to be an easier concept that can be defined using objective terms. It would be a mistake, however, to think that competence is limited to the observation of a person's ability to perform certain tasks. A sense of competence is just as dynamic as the sense of identity and occupational therapists need to recognise.

- how competence links to occupational identity
- how competence links to the impact of the environment

Links to occupational identity

Just as occupational identity is more than role identity, necessitating a synthesised understanding of roles and relationships and the person's volition in the context of the environment, occupational competence is more than how well a person is able to perform certain tasks, activities, or occupations. The person's performance must also be regarded in relation to his or her identity. In this way, occupational

DOI: 10.4324/9781003046301-6

competence becomes 'the ability to actualise a desired occupational identity in a way that provides satisfaction' (Bar and Jarus 2015, p6045). In other words,

> *'Occupational competence is the degree to which one sustains a successful pattern of occupational participation that reflects one's occupational identity.... Thus, while identity has to do with the subjective meaning of one's occupational life, competence has to do with putting that identity into action in an ongoing way'*

(de las Heras de Pablo et al. 2017a, p117)

This means that, even when occupational therapists seek to assess a person's performance through direct observation, the occupations being observed should be ones that the person needs to, wants to, or is expected to do (Polatajko et al. 2000). Improved occupational performance goes hand in hand with improved participation in life situations that are personally relevant and meaningful (Verhoef et al. 2014). By implication, therefore, one cannot measure a person's performance unless one has already gained an understanding of the person's identity. Only then can one assess whether the person is following through their chosen occupations and performing them to a certain standard, and then begin to compare the objective reality with the person's subjective experience (see Table 6.1).

Links to environmental impact

In addition to viewing performance in relation to occupational identity, understanding a person's overall competence involves situating performance in its environmental context. Competence encompasses a person's ability to meet environmental demands (Bar and Jarus 2015) and the two are interrelated, with competence being influenced or even governed by the demands and constraints of the current environment (Yerxa 1991) (see Table 6.1).

The various environments frequented by the person may either promote or inhibit occupational competence (Rogers 1982), and both the positive and the negative qualities of these environments must be represented when attempting to describe a person's occupational competence. An outline of a person's occupational competence might, therefore, include references to the compensatory supports that might be in place, such as the level of personal support received, the provision of assistive technologies, and the impact of medication (Sandell et al. 2013), as well as the influence of policies and procedures (Murad et al. 2013), and the opportunities afforded by the physical space.

Table 6.1 Comparing the identity and competence sections

Identity	Competence
• Represents the person's *subjective* viewpoint	• Describes *objective* information
• Roots the person's identity in their *past*	• Focuses on *present* circumstances

Box 6.1 Author's note

by Dr Rob Brooks

The traditional report formats used by occupational therapists tend to focus on a person's performance in a range of everyday tasks. Sadly, this is too often the result of process-driven systems in which the occupational therapist assesses predetermined activities such as washing, dressing, cooking, budgeting, travel, etc., without considering what the person wants or needs to do. One of the things that I love about occupational formulation is its ability to cut through any pre-set expectations and focus instead on the needs and wishes of the individual:

- if the person was involved in a motorbike accident, then the therapist will need to assess the impact on the person's skills
- if the same person has a role as a tattoo artist, then the therapist will need to have a sense of their ability in this profession
- if the person also has an interest in scuba-diving, then the therapist will need to understand whether this constitutes a regular part of their routine and,
- if this person owns a pet snake and has been admitted to hospital, the therapist will need to know who is looking after the snake

In other words, the competence section encourages the therapist to review the person's skills, abilities, routines, and environmental contexts in relation to their roles, relationships, life turning points, and interests. In my experience, this stimulates a fuller and more person-centred assessment, leading to more effective interventions that are more meaningful for the person ... as well as being more satisfying for the therapist.

Including strengths and limitations

Key to formulating a person's occupational competence is the ability to conceptualise strengths and limitations (Kielhofner and Forsyth 2008). Whereas a medical diagnosis might indicate impairment, an occupational formulation must record functional abilities as well as functional disabilities (Rogers 1982). Indeed, even when the problems are foremost in the mind the individual and others may be focusing on the person's difficulties, it is essential that occupational therapists demonstrate their hope and positive expectation by bringing to people's attention any assets that can be built upon.

The importance of a hopeful perspective was famously articulated by Reilly (1962) when she promoted Occupational Therapy as one of the great ideas of 20th- century medicine. According to Reilly, the profession is based on an 'optimistic view' of human nature – one that finds positive resources and potential in every human being. This does not mean that occupational therapists are naive or unrealistic. The strengths that they notice, however small they might be, do exist. They seek only to counter the prevailing emphasis on pathology by illuminating a person's existing skills and capacities while still identifying any weaknesses that might be alleviated or reduced (Yerxa 1991).

Box 6.2   Author's note

by Sue Parkinson

Although people are usually referred to Occupational Therapy when they are experiencing significant difficulties – typically affecting their ability to participate in various occupations and often leading to less fulfilling routines – this should never blind a therapist to the individual's strengths or positives in their situation. Everyone has their strengths, and because occupational competence depends upon a person's myriad skills and wide-ranging environmental contexts, I am convinced that a therapist can always find something positive to comment on. For example,

- a person may struggle to make friends, but is still able to co-operate with others; or
- a person experiences problems at work but has already taken certain steps to resolve this; or
- a person may have difficulties bathing independently but benefits from having various aids and adaptations

Competence and the Model of Human Occupation

In the Model of Human Occupation (ed. Taylor 2017), occupational competence and occupational identity are interrelated (Phelan and Kinsella 2009) in so much as competence in the performance of activities helps to shape a person's identity (Christiansen 1999) and the fulfilment of a positive identity guides a person's participation in occupations. Over time, the person then develops skills and the ability to perform these occupations with ease, and this is known as occupational competence (O'Brien and Kielhofner [posthumous] 2017). Indeed, the concept of occupational competence in the Model of Human occupation only exists in relation to occupational identity, in that it is 'the degree to which one sustains a successful pattern of occupational participation that reflects one's identity' (de las Heras de Pablo et al. 2017a, p117).

Once a therapist has gained an idea of an individual's occupational identity, the Model of Human Occupation (ed. Taylor 2017) goes on to provide detailed directions for gauging how well the person's occupational competence matches their identity (see Figure 6.1). It manages to do this through a comprehensive range of assessments that enrich and deepen a therapist's understanding of how a person's *skills, routines, performance, and environment* support occupational competence (see Table 6.2).

Routines

In addition to being able to demonstrate a range of skills, occupational competence means integrating basic responsibilities and role obligations into a satisfying lifestyle, in which routines may be evident on a daily, weekly, monthly, seasonal or annual basis. The Model of Human Occupation supports the analysis of a person's

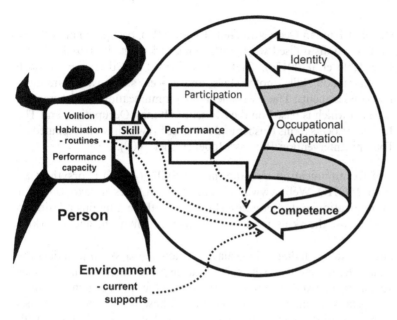

Figure 6.1 MOHO concepts that contribute to a sense of competence.
(Source: image adapted from Kielhofner's MOHO textbook (ed. Taylor 2017).

Table 6.2 Basic content of an occupational competence section

How
• Routines
• Skills
• Abilities (how well the person performs activities); and
• Current environmental contexts match the person's identity

habitual use of time through a number of assessments, most notably the Occupational Performance History Interview (Kielhofner et al. 2004).

The Occupational Performance History Interview, Version 2.1 (OPHI-II) (Kielhofner et al. 2004) is available from MOHO Web (www.moho.uic.edu) and supports therapists to assess occupational competence with regards to whether an individual currently

• maintains a satisfying lifestyle
• fulfils role obligations
• works toward goals
• meets personal performance standards
• organises time for responsibilities
• participates in interests

Skills

According to the Model of Human Occupation (ed. Taylor 2017), occupational skills are observable, goal-directed actions utilised when performing tasks, activities, and occupations (de las Heras de Pablo et al. 2017a). They can be divided into three types of skill (communication and interaction skills, motor skills, and process skills) which are identified and defined in two assessments: The Assessment of Communication and Interaction Skills (Forsyth et al. 1998) which is based on the Model of Human Occupation, and The Assessment of Motor and Process Skills (Fisher and Jones 2014) which is underpinned by the Occupational Therapy Intervention Process Model (Fisher 2009).

The Assessment of Communication and Interaction Skills (ACIS) (Forsyth et al. 1998) (available from MOHO Web www.moho.uic.edu) provides a taxonomy for conceptualising communication and interaction skills across three domains relating to a person's non-verbal skills, the skills used to exchange information, and the skills necessary for relating to others.

It itemises 20 skills in total, including 'Physicality' (or non-verbal skills) including the use of gaze to communicate, the use of gestures for enhancing communication, as well as the use of posture to convey non-verbal messages. Thereafter, the 'Information exchange' section assesses how a person maintains a conversation and how vocal expression assists interaction. Finally, the 'Relations' section focuses on such skills as collaborating with others, conforming to social norms, establishing rapport, and respecting the needs of others.

The Assessment of Motor and Process Skills (AMPS) (Fisher and Jones 2014) is a powerful, occupation-based assessment (see https://www.innovativeotsolutions.com). Certification in this assessment allows occupational therapists to measures a person's ability to perform activities of daily living by rating 16 motor skills and 20 process skills.

Motor skills examine a person's ability to maintain a functional posture, produce flowing movements, and exercise appropriate strength and effort when completing everyday tasks. Process skills are concerned with the person's ability to be goal-directed and ability to work through tasks in an organised fashion by maintaining focussed attention, using objects appropriately, and modifying their actions in response to environmental cues.

Performance

Further assessments based on the Model of Human Occupation (available from MOHO Web www.moho.uic.edu) can be used to gain a detailed understanding of how a person performs particular activities.

The Occupational Self Assessment (OSA) (Baron et al. 2006) which is now available in a shortened version (Popova et al. 2019) elicits information about a person's performance when 'taking care of myself', 'getting where I need to go', 'managing my finances', and 'managing my basic needs (food, medicine)', and other everyday activities.

The School Setting Interview (Hemmingsson et al. 2005) can be used with children to investigate how well they do mathematics, do homework and take exams, or participate in sports activities, practical subjects, the classroom as a whole, or social activities during breaks, etc.

The Volitional Questionnaire (VQ) (de las Heras et al. 2007) captures a person's inner motivation by noticing their intentions and does not set out to assess how well a person completes any particular activity. However, the fact that it is an observational assessment allows a therapist to record empirical data based on whether a person

* shows curiosity
* initiates actions/tasks
* tries new things
* shows preferences
* shows that an activity is special or significant
* stays engaged
* indicates goals
* shows pride
* tries to solve problems
* tries to correct mistakes
* pursues an activity to completion/accomplishment
* invests additional energy/emotion/attention
* seeks/accepts additional responsibilities
* seeks/accepts challenges

Environment

According to the Model of Human Occupation, the environment influences a person's skills, performance, and participation by providing opportunities and resources as well as demands and constraints (Fisher et al. 2017). When analysing occupational competence, therapists must take the impact of the environment into account and consider whether the person's immediate or local environment is supporting or restricting occupational competence. Two assessments assist this task: the Occupational Performance History Interview (Kielhofner et al. 2004) and the Residential Environment Impact Scale (Fisher et al. 2014) (both available from MOHO Web www.moho.uic.edu).

The Occupational Performance History Interview, Second Version (OPHI-II) (Kielhofner et al. 2004) aids therapists to place a person's competence in the context of various occupational behaviour settings, relating to the person's major productive roles, leisure interests, and home life. In each case, the therapist takes note of the influence exerted by the social group, the occupational demands, and the impact of the physical space and the objects within the space.

The Residential Environment Impact Scale (REIS) (Fisher et al. 2014) is a consulting instrument that has been designed to examine the impact of community residential facilities. It prompts therapists to study the impact of the environment under four separate headings

* *everyday space*: accessibility, adequacy, homelike qualities, sensory qualities, and visual supports
* *everyday objects*: availability, adequacy, homelike qualities, physical attributes, and variety of objects

- *enabling relationships*: availability of people and how they enable respect, support & facilitation, provision of information, and empowerment
- *structure of activity*: activity and time demands, the appeal of activities, impact of routines, and opportunities for decision making

An awareness of the above assessments provides therapists with invaluable evidence as to whether a person has the skills to perform activities, how well these activities are performed, how often, and with what degree of support. Taken together, this information can be used to demonstrate the degree to which the person's occupational competence complements their established occupational identity (see Table 6.3 - Top tips for the Occupational Competence section).

Table 6.3 Top tips for the Occupational Competence section

- As before, when writing the Occupational Identity section, write this section in a user-friendly way

  o Avoid using technical language
  o Start and end the section with positives
  o End a sentence with the person's strengths if the sentences refer to both their strengths and their limitations

- Aim to offer answers to all the questions that a reader might have after reading the Identity section, regarding what is actually happening
- For each experience mentioned in the identity section, follow up with *objective* information regarding what the person can or cannot do, what they are required to do, how often they do things, when they last did them, who with, where and with what level of support
- Try to follow through each experience in the same order that they were mentioned in the identity section
- It may not be necessary to comment on the person's competence in relation to past turning points, unless it is worth noting how well they are coping
- Focus as much as possible on current circumstances and only refer to the person's history when the person's strengths are best represented by past successes
- State the limitations *and* the strengths that the person possesses, in terms of their skills, abilities, routines, and environmental contexts
- Resist the temptation to refer to whether the person is following through any previously agreed treatment plans, as the formulation marks a fresh start. Also, the competence section must reflect how the person's competence matches their long-standing occupational identity, and most people do not identify themselves primarily as clients, patients, or service users
- Avoid giving the person's viewpoint in this section. Record empirical observations rather than offering analysis or making any judgements
- Rather than saying that a person has 'difficulty with' or 'struggles with' an activity (phrases which might represent the person's *subjective* viewpoint), justify these statements by describing their behaviour and what actually happens
- Do not state that the person is 'confident' or 'anxious' or 'motivated'. These statements relate to the person's feelings, which should have been recorded in the identity section. Instead, use this section to describe the person's behaviours, i.e., the impact of their anxiety or confidence or motivation on their skills and performance
- Do not assume the reader will know that the person is able to perform everyday self-care activities or that they have good communication and interaction, process skills, and motor skills

Box 6.3 Author's note

by Sue Parkinson

While the identity section should be acceptable to the person, because it represents their own viewpoint, it should also be possible for the person to acknowledge the objective nature of the information in the competence section. So you will need to be careful about including anything that cannot be justified by your own observation and it is recommended that you acknowledge when information comes from other sources. For example, you might start a sentence with phrases indicating that the person's *family* have noticed a particular behaviour, or that the person's *employer* has commented on an element of the person's performance.

It is crucial is to avoid offering explanations for aspects of the person's competence - both because such explanations may not be accepted by the person and because it may suggest that nothing can be changed. For instance,

- If the person believes that they are destined to save the universe and does not believe that they are ill, then this information is rightly included in the identity section as it represents their subjective viewpoint. When it comes to following up this information in the competence section, it would be unhelpful simply to say that the person is wrong, but the therapist might be able to identify an objective consequence that the person can accept – e.g., that voicing this belief has led to disagreements with various family members
- If the person is staying in bed for most of the day, then their reasoning should already have been noted in the identity section. Perhaps they feel that they do not have any energy or that there is nothing worth getting up for. In the competence section, stating that the person stays in bed due to their 'reduced motivation' or their 'anxiety' may serve to vindicate or rationalise their inactivity

In my opinion, the beauty of creating a formulation consisting of two sections that mirror each other, and where both are indisputable in their own way, is that the analysis is not overt. Analysis can always be challenged, whereas the formulation tolerates different perspectives. It is open to interpretation and yet those involved still manage to perceive the way forward by comparing and contrasting the two halves (see Figure 6.2).

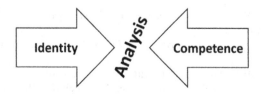

Figure 6.2 Analysis is not overt.

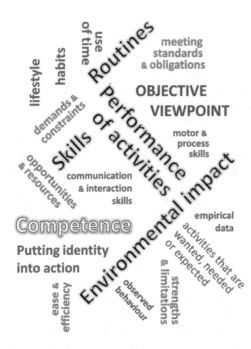

Figure 6.3 Occupational competence.

References

Bar MA, Jarus T (2015) The effect of engagement in everyday occupations, role overload and social support on health and life satisfaction among mothers. *International Journal of Environmental Research and Public Health, 12(6)*, 6045–6065.

Baron K, Kielhofner G, Iyenger A, Goldhammer V, Wolenski J, (2006) *A User's Manual for the Occupational Self Assessment (OSA), Version 2.2.* Chicago, University of Illinois.

Christiansen CH (1999) Defining lives: occupation as identity: an essay on competence, coherence and the creation of meaning. *American Journal of Occupational Therapy, 53(6)*, 547–558.

de las Heras, CG, Geist, R, Kielhofner, G, Li Y (2007) *A user's Guide to the Volitional Questionnaire (VQ). Version 4.1.* Chicago, University of Illinois.

de las Heras de Pablo, Fan C-W, Kielhofner G [posthumous] (2017a) Dimensions of Doing. In RR Taylor, ed. *Kielhofner's Model of Human Occupation: Theory and Application.* Philadelphia: Wolters Kluwer. 107–122.

Fisher AG (2009) *Occupational Therapy Intervention Process Model: A Model for Planning and Implementing Top–Down, Client-Centered, and Occupation-Based Interventions.* Ft. Collins, CO: Three Star Press.

Fisher G, Forsyth K, Harrison M et al. (2014) *Residential Environment Impact Scale (REIS) Version 4.0.* Chicago: University of Illinois.

Fisher AG, Jones KB (2014) *Assessment of Motor and Process Sskills.* Vol 2: User manual (8th ed.) Fort Collins, CO: Three Stars Press

Fisher G, Parkinson S, Haglund L (2017) The environment and human occupation. In: Taylor R, ed., *Kielhofner's Model of Human Occupation.* 5th ed. Philadelphia: Wolters Kluwer. 91–106.

Forsyth K, Salamy M, Simon S, Kielhofner G (1998) *The Assessment of Communication and Interaction Skills (ACIS) Version 4.0.* Chicago: University of Illinois.

Hemmingsson H, Egilson S, Hoffman O, Kielhofner G (2005) *The School Setting Interview (SSI) Version 3.0.* Chicago: University of Illinois.

Kielhofner G, Forsyth K (2008) Occupational engagement: how clients achieve change. In: G Kielhofner ed. *Model of Human Occupation: theory and application.* 4th ed. Baltimore: Lippincott, Williams & Wilkins, 101–109.

Kielhofner G, Mallinson T, Crawford C, Nowak M, Rigby M, Henry A, Walens D (2004) *Occupational Performance History Interview (OPHI-II), Version 2.1.* Chicago: University of Illinois.

Murad MS, O'Brien L, Farnworth L, Chien C-W (2013) Occupational competence and its relationship to emotional health in injured workers in return to work programs: a Malaysian study. *Scandinavian Journal of Occupational Therapy, 20*(2), 101–110.

O'Brien JC, Kielhofner G [posthumous] (2017) The interaction between the person and the environment. In: RR Taylor ed., *Kielhofner's Model of Human Occupation.* 5th ed. Philadelphia: Wolters Kluwer. 24–37.

Phelan S, Kinsella EA (2009) Occupational Identity: engaging socio-cultural perspectives. *Journal of Occupational Science, 16*(2), 85–91.

Polatajko HJ (1992) Naming and framing Occupational Therapy: a lecture dedicated to the life of Nancy B. *Canadian Journal of Occupational Therapy, 59*(4), 189–199.

Polatajko HJ, Mandich A, Martini R (2000). Dynamic performance analysis: a framework for understanding occupational performance. *American Journal of Occupational Therapy, 54*(1), 65–72.

Popova ES, Ostrowski RK, Wescott JJ, Taylor RR (2019) Development and validation of the occupational self assessment–short form. *American Journal of Occupational Therapy, 73*(3).

Reilly M (1962) Occupational Therapy can be one of the great ideas of 20th century medicine. *American Journal of Occupational Therapy 16*(1), 1–9.

Rogers JC (1982) Order and disorder in Occupational Therapy. *American Journal of Occupational Therapy, 36*(1), 29–35.

Sandell C, Kjellberg A, Taylor R (2013) Participating in diagnostic experience: adults with neuropsychiatric disorders. *Scandinavian Journal of Occupational Therapy, 20*(2), 136–142.

Taylor RR ed. (2017) *Kielhofner's Model of Human Occupation.* 5th ed. Philadelphia: Wolters Kluwer.

Verhoef JAC, Roebroeck ME, van Schaardenburgh N, Floothuis MCSG, Miedema HS (2014) Improved occupational performance of young adults with a physical disability after a vocational rehabilitation intervention. *Journal of Occupational Rehabilitation, 24*(1), 42–45.

Yerxa EJ (1991) Seeking a relevant, ethical and realistic way of knowing Occupational Therapy. *American Journal of Occupational Therapy, 45*(3), 199–204.

7 Determining the key issues for occupational adaptation

When an occupational therapist has a sense of a person's identity and a sense of how the person's competence matches this identity, the next stage of the formulation process is to establish the key issues that will encapsulate the focus for the planned therapy. This focus is often regarded as being the central feature of Occupational Therapy. For example, Mary Law et al. (1998) wrote that *'The uniqueness of occupational therapy lies in its focus on occupation as central in promoting and maintaining health and well-being'* (p82).

As such, when the key issues are being considered, care must be taken to ensure that they encompass the person's occupational needs. The identity and competence sections now serve as the 'back story' – setting the scene at the beginning of the story and developing the themes in the middle of the story – and the issues are likely to stem either from the interests and goals outlined in the identity section or from the limitations that are apparent in the competence section. The key issues guide how the story ends by articulating the occupations that are key for the person's future health and well-being.

Defining the nature of occupation

Occupational therapy promotes health and well-being through occupation (World Federation of Occupational Therapists 2012), but what exactly is an occupational issue? Simply put, occupations refer to everyday tasks undertaken as part of an individual's lifestyle (Golledge 1998), however, there is no consensus on a universal definition of occupation (Leclair 2010). Instead, a multi-layering of related explanations is required to obtain a rich understanding of this vital endeavour. It has been referred to as goal-directed doing (Gray 1997) or what people do when they occupy themselves by 'looking after themselves (*self-care*), enjoying life (*leisure*), and contributing to the social and economic fabric of their communities' (*productivity*) (Canadian Association of Occupational Therapists [CAOT] 2017). The concepts of self-care, leisure, and productivity occur repeatedly under different guises and have been referred to as activities of daily living, play, and work (Taylor and Kielhofner [posthumous] 2017) as well as self-maintenance, relaxation/entertainment/creativity/celebration, and productive pursuits (Christiansen et al. 2005).

All the above domains are culturally defined and are seen to exist within a temporal, physical and sociocultural context (Taylor and Kielhofner 2017) – at a certain time, in certain places and with certain people. Individuals participate in them over extended periods of time because the occupations are personally and culturally meaningful

DOI: 10.4324/9781003046301-7

(Mackey and Nancarrow 2006). Moreover, in addition to enabling individuals to connect with what is meaningful and allowing social interaction between people, they also provide the mechanism for social development at a community, national and international level (Wilcock 2006). Put like this, the magnitude of the universal significance of occupation is truly awe-inspiring.

Recognising the impact of genericism

At this point, it should be acknowledged that the significance of occupation is sometimes underrated, and the pressure to work within a reductionist, biomedical, or generic paradigm means that occupational therapy practice has not always adhered to its founding principles (Leclair 2010). This state of affairs was first perceived as a threat to the occupational therapy profession in the late 1970s, when it was recognised that occupational therapists were losing sight of the meaning of occupation (Kielhofner 1992). The resulting crisis brought about a re-emergence of an occupation-focused paradigm (Whiteford et al. 2000) – with conceptual frameworks and models emphasising the occupational nature of human beings – along with the identification of research evidence that supported the relationship between occupation, health, and well-being (Law et al. 1998).

Despite the shared vision within a profession that is committed to holding occupation at its core (Pettican and Bryant 2007) ... despite the research evidence to support the centrality of occupation (Law et al. 1998) ... despite the development of conceptual models to support the move away from a reductionist stance (Joosten 2015) ... and despite warnings that occupational therapy is at risk if occupational therapists do not focus on occupation (Poulden and Oke 1990, Gustafsson et al. 2014, Joosten 2015), occupational therapists have continued to focus on impairment as much as, if not more than, occupation (Di Tommaso et al. 2016). These concerns are summarised by Pettican and Bryant (2007) in the following statement:

> *'The trend for occupational therapists to perform a predominantly generic role ... has been an area of discussion over recent years, with concerns focusing primarily on the potential loss of core skills and, ultimately, of professional identity'* (p140)

This pull towards generic or reductionist roles has been prevalent for decades, both in mental health services (Pettican and Bryant 2007) and in physical health services. Back in 1998, Gray was disheartened to find that occupational therapists working in physical health services were focusing on isolated aspects of performance rather than meaningful occupation. They were selecting purposeful or even non-purposeful repetitive activities to improve the person's biomechanical impairments, using equipment and tasks that were unrelated to a person's everyday experience. It was assumed that changing the various performance components would automatically lead to enhanced occupational outcomes, albeit that occupation is based on a complex dynamic interaction with the environment that cannot be predicted on performance capacity alone.

In 2001, Pierre noted that an occupational focus was valued by Swedish occupational therapists working in a geriatric clinic but was often not overtly referred to in their documentation. Later, in 2016, Di Tommaso and her colleagues reported that occupational therapists working in a range of Australian services had difficulty articulating how they used occupation in practice. The occupational therapists had been qualified for no more than 6 years and many of them chose to use *impairment-focused* interventions even though they recognised the motivational value of *occupation-based* practice. This approach was rationalised on the basis that clients needed to regain their performance abilities before they could participate in occupations. It appeared that many occupational therapists found it difficult to harness occupation in their workplaces and may have resorted to using impairment-focused exercises and strategies as a means towards the end goal of occupational participation. The trouble with this plan, especially when progress towards the end goal is not measured, is that the means come to be seen as ends in their own right.

Box 7.1   Author's note

by Sue Parkinson

When I teach occupational formulation, I invariably ask the participants what they hope to gain from the teaching session. Many are hoping to discover a more concise way to communicate the focus of occupational therapy, but their overriding concern is how to make their communication convincing and compelling so that they can maximise their profession-specific practice. Some are able to offer occupational interventions but fear that their importance is disregarded, while others recognise that their interventions are moving further and further away from their occupational roots.

Reasserting an occupational focus

Anne Fisher (2013) made an important distinction between being occupation-centred, occupation-focused, and occupation-based:

- occupation-centred refers to the perspective in which occupation is deemed to be at the philosophical core of the profession and services of occupational therapy
- occupation-based refers to the act of engaging a person in an occupation for the purposes of intervention and evaluation
- occupation-focused refers to the focussed attention on occupation which might involve gathering information about occupations, identifying occupational priorities, negotiating occupational goals, as well – it can be inferred – as constructing occupational formulations

She concludes that occupational therapists must implement occupation-based 'and/or' occupation-focused methods if they are to remain occupation-centred. In fact, it would be hard to be occupation-based without being occupation-focused, as occupational choices involve 'deliberation' and 'commitment', and require information-gathering, reflection, and the consideration of imagined possibilities and alternatives (Kielhofner 2008, p15). Without occupation-focused reflection, occupational therapists would risk offering and making *activity* choices rather than *occupational* choices – ones that might be necessary but would have a short-term impact (*ibid*).

Box 7.2   Author's note

by Dr Rob Brooks

Early in my career, I remember being incredibly impressed by The Well Elderly study (Jackson et al. 1998) when it was first published, and its use of occupation-focused interventions has had a lasting impact on my professional reasoning. The study investigated an innovative occupational programme known as Lifestyle Redesign as part of a Randomised Controlled Trial, and I realised that the programme consisted of occupation-focused elements (taught presentations, peer exchange, and personal exploration) as well as occupation-based elements (direct experience of occupation). It was compared with two control groups: one which was provided with a social activities programme led by staff who were not occupational therapists, and one which received no treatment. All were assessed using a comprehensive battery of measures and those receiving the occupational therapy programme made significantly greater gains, or fewer losses, than participants in either of the control groups. Jackson and her colleagues concluded that the success of Lifestyle Redesign had important implications and 'were contrary to the cliché that "keeping busy keeps you healthy"' (p334). It is true that the social activities provided to one of the control groups were more *activity*-based than *occupation*-based, but the achievements of Lifestyle Redesign were certainly attributed to the more invisible, occupation-focused aspects of the programme, including a focus on and sensitivity to personal and cultural meaningfulness.

According to Gray (1998), occupations must have context, possess meaningfulness to the individual, and hold a degree of purposefulness or goal-directedness. Purposefulness on its own is insufficient and this means that everyday self-care activities such as washing and dressing, which are often classed as occupations, lose their therapeutic impact if not valued by the individual. Likewise, engaging people in exercises to practise certain behaviours does not constitute occupation-based practise, although Gray acknowledged that these exercises might be used in preparation for and in conjunction with occupation.

Greber (2018) went a step further than Gray, in urging occupational therapists to resist the tendency to promote a particular way of working while decrying the other. He recognised that the call for occupation-centred practice may have given occupational therapists a voice to assert their unique skills, but it may also have undermined occupational therapy practice in places where mechanistic and generic strategies were valued. Therefore, he deduced that

'Our profession must embrace a pluralistic narrative rather than an absolutist stance thinly disguised as an extreme relativist one' (p71)

A pluralist stance suggests that therapists should appreciate and integrate a continuum of perspectives and practices that arise from a genuine concern to enhance occupational performance. It does not mean that occupation-based practice or occupation-focused practice should be abandoned completely; merely that generic strategies and interventions should be tolerated, incorporated, and maybe even embraced, especially when retaining occupation-based practice is limited by a competitive, medical-oriented market. However, this leaves occupational therapists with a dilemma: how do occupational therapists preserve any sense of their occupation-centredness? Once again, clinicians and theorists emphasise the importance of maintaining an occupation-focused stance in which the distinct professional viewpoint is articulated. Gillen and Greber (2014) point out that

> '*Whilst, as occupational therapists, our practice must conform to the pragmatic constraints of a service, our potential to talk in occupation-focused ways is unrestrained*' (p40)

More importantly, the constraints of a service do not restrict a therapist's ability to *think* in an occupation focused way, and this might be the most important skill of all. Turner and Alsop understood this when they wrote about the unique core skills of occupational therapists in 2015. They argued that in order to try and make the occupational therapy profession more visible and clearly understood, it was the complex invisible skills that merited further attention. Their opinion was influenced by the work of Mattingly (1994) who observed that the skill of the occupational therapist lies in framing and reframing the problem area. They concluded that

> '*The unique core skills of occupational therapists are largely unseen. They are the reasoning skills used to apply the understanding of occupation and its impact on health to the meaningful activities and occupations of service users. Visible practice skills are diverse and some may be shared with other professions. While some activities can appear mundane, forming the rationale for their use is the unique core skill of occupational therapists*'

(Turner and Alsop 2015, p739)

Forming the rationale for interventions is surely the purpose of occupational formulation – whether the formulation exists solely in the therapists' mind, or whether it takes shape in how they verbalise their reasoning, or whether it is written down in a formal document.

Box 7.3   Author's note

by Sue Parkinson

When working with occupational therapists to determine the occupational focus and ultimate basis of therapy, I frequently encounter individuals who find it difficult to switch from a generic mindset because they have become used to formulating treatment plans that focus on 'decreased anxiety', or 'increased standing tolerance', or 'reduced alcohol intake', or 'improved sensory processing'. In these circumstances, I challenge them to think about the person's motivation for working towards these aims: *what will the person be able to do if these aims were achieved?* I also acknowledge that when negotiating the key issues with some people, one might accept a more generic/pluralist focus if (a) the occupational therapist is expected to perform a generic role, or (b) the individuals themselves are so preoccupied with managing the immediate problems that they feel unable to think about their future occupations – what they want or need to do.

More than this, I remind the therapists that framing an issue using occupational language does not prevent them from recommending or facilitating generic interventions. For instance, you could help a mother to care for her baby *and* facilitate anxiety management as part of this process, or you could help an older person to re-engage in their domestic activities *and* promote exercise designed to increase their range of movement. Ultimately, however, one measures the *occupational* impact.

I wonder how many occupational therapists frame their treatment plans using generic terms because these have more status or acceptance in the multi-disciplinary workforce? My belief is that the focus on ordinary, everyday occupations will have more credence when they are supported by compelling evidence regarding the person's sense of identity and competence. The issues on their own may have little weight with those who are yet to grasp the power of the ordinary and the commonplace, which is why it helps if the occupational therapist can bring the person's story to life with a well-crafted formulation that articulates the rationale for an occupational focus.

Embracing occupational language

Craig Greber (2018) suggested that occupational report headings may represent the first step towards adopting occupation-focused practice. He echoed the views of Ilott and Mounter (2000) who recommended using occupational terminology to educate others about the merits and values of occupational therapy. This viewpoint also fits nicely with the recommendation of Poulden and Oke (1990) that occupational therapists should decide upon a single contribution, however small, that might take occupational therapy forward into the future. Could this decision lead to occupational therapists choosing to instigate occupational formulations that embrace occupational language?

Using occupational language is a small action that is thought to play a vital role in highlighting the role of occupational therapists in the multi-disciplinary team. At a managerial or political level, this may include terminology drawn from occupational science, calling for 'occupational justice' (Wilcock and Townsend 2000) to rectify 'occupational deprivation' (Whiteford et al. 2000), redress 'occupational imbalance', or remedy 'occupational alienation' (Townsend and Wilcock 2004). However, clinicians must also be mindful of using language that can be understood by service users (Brown and Bourke-Taylor 2012) in order to assist their understanding of the role of occupational therapy and to strengthen their commitment (Gillen and Greber 2014).

If occupational therapists are to use accessible occupational language to enhance people's understanding of the purpose of therapy, perhaps the greatest impact can be made when negotiating an intervention plan. Occupational therapists usually become involved in a person's care when the person experiences a transition which necessitates adjustment and adaptation (Blair 2000)t, and at such times the individual is often acutely aware of changes to their environment, motivation, roles, routines, habits, skills, performance, and participation. In these circumstances, occupational therapists can provide individuals, and their families and carers, with a language in which to explore and begin to remedy these issues. Understanding can then lead to more realistic goal-setting (Di Tommaso et al. 2016), which, rather than focusing solely on the performance of short-term activity-based interventions, focuses on the participation of the person in long-term occupations.

Instead of the goal of therapy being 'sensory regulation', 'stress management', or 'standing tolerance', occupational therapists need to focus on which occupations the person will be able to participate in once the various strategies, techniques, and exercises have made a difference. Even some much-used phrases by occupational therapists, such as 'daily structure' or 'balanced routine', do little to convey what the person will actually do to fill their time. This might be riding a bike, or making friends, or finding a job, or being able to look after oneself – whatever the person aspires to do (see Table 7.1) Simply put, writing occupation-focused goals requires occupational therapists to explicitly focus on the 'in order to do what' component of therapy (Pereira 2015, p208), and Joosten (2015) argues that this need not be a time-consuming process:

'*In the time it takes to set and write a goal with a client about increasing hand strength or range of movement, we can equally write a goal about being able to grasp a spoon and eat dinner or hold a hand of cards …. To document that someone showered safely and independently while standing for 10 minutes, presents a very different picture of our intervention, and our unique contribution, than reporting improved balance …. Reporting that a client was discharged and had returned to work with a wheelchair that enabled independent mobility, rather than documenting 'she was discharged with wheelchair', reflects a knowing of our clients and a focus on their return to desired occupational roles and contexts*' (p221)

The issues identified in the formulation process will provide the central focus in subsequent goals, yet it has been noted that occupational therapists may engage in 'self-limiting practices' when writing goals (Pereira 2015) - often by narrowing goals to the short-term objectives or targets that might be achieved within the intervention setting. Gray challenged this practice in 1998 and advanced the viewpoint that occupational therapists are best placed to see beyond the short-term gains that might be made within a healthcare setting to the over-arching goals for each person. These take place within the person's own environment and naturally extend to 'personally satisfying organised daily routines of culturally relevant activities: occupation' (p357). In this way,

Table 7.1 Examples of occupational and non-occupational issues

Occupational issues regarding skills performance and participation	*Non-occupational issues (i.e., symptom management, increasing capacity and prescribed interventions)*
• Meeting new people • Reaching for objects • Developing new roles • Riding a bike	• Anxiety management • Range of movement • Bereavement counselling • Sensory integration

'Everything that is done in occupational therapy evaluation and treatment should be directed toward the ultimate outcome of restoring client's [sic] "occupational lives." Therapists are called upon to analyze not only a client's performance of given occupations, but also his or her overall use of time, daily habits and routines, activities in relation to the developmental continuum, and need as an occupational being for creativity, competence, and challenge'

(Gray 1998, p357)

Box 7.4 Author's note

by Dr Rob Brooks

When thinking about the problems that arise when reducing a meaningful occupation to its constituent parts, the following example often comes to mind. It involves a person whose most heartfelt wish is to find a soulmate – a girlfriend or a boyfriend – which is perhaps one of the most natural ambitions that a person can have. However, the occupational therapist decides to reduce the goal to something that is more manageable – perhaps because their time with the person is limited, or perhaps because they fear that the person's goal is unobtainable, or perhaps because they do not know how to break the person's dream into smaller goals. They, therefore, decide to encourage the person to take small steps towards finding a partner, and begin by setting the objective of 'having regular showers'! Although it would be easy enough to set measurable targets for having regular showers, this plan is almost bound to fail because

- the therapist has imposed their own values onto the situation and the person's wishes have been ignored, leading to disaffection with the therapy process
- having regular showers does not automatically lead to finding a soulmate, and may be irrelevant
- by trying to avoid a goal that might lead to failure, the therapist has already suggested that failure is expected

Of course, writing long-term goals that extend beyond the confines of a health service and beyond the expected timeframe for therapy is perfectly possible. Similarly, writing an aspirational goal that may never be met is easy enough. The challenge is how to write sub-goals that link perfectly with the long-term goal and yet can be met in the short-term. Chapter 9 will explain how this can be achieved and how therapists can negotiate goals even when success is uncertain. The method described is based on the principle that practitioners can never guarantee a particular outcome. Instead, their role is to see how far they can take a person towards their eventual goals. The only restriction is that the goals should support occupational participation in society and be legal. So, although a keen interest is taken in how a person's sense of identity and competence are shaped by 'dark occupations' (Twinley 2013), which are typically antisocial or unhealthy to some extent, the key issues should focus on pro-social occupations that enable health and well-being.

Occupational issues and the Model of Human Occupation

The Model of Human Occupation has always been regarded as an *occupation focused* model – one that focuses on issues related to occupational adaptation rather than 'the remediation of a set of symptoms or impairments' (Taylor and Kielhofner [posthumous] 2017, p6). In addition to referring to occupation as 'work, play, or activities of daily living' (*ibid*), the model states that everything that a person does can be broken down into various levels of participation, of which there are three major levels:

- *performance skills* required for occupational performance (requiring occupation-based observation of communication and interaction skills, and motor and process skills)
- *performance* of activities (requiring occupation-based observations of how well a person performs a task or activity), and ultimately
- *participation* in occupation (which benefits from occupation-based observations of how a person spends their time and their volitional behaviours, but also requires occupation-focused enquiries regarding the person's subjective experience)

These levels were further sub-divided by Carmen de las Heras de Pablo et al. (2017a, 2017b) (see Figure 7.1) They stated that the first phase of role development happens when people explore or experience what might be expected of them and the skills that are demanded of them, before practising the various steps and tasks required in activities or the participation of roles (de las Heras de Pablo 2017b). These ideas built on her work to promote occupational participation (2011) and are elaborated on in the Remotivation Process (de las Heras et al. 2019). Together they demonstrate the scope and depth of practice undertaken by occupational therapists. Although role development may be the ultimate goal, all the stages have their importance and may be identified as an occupational issue depending on the needs of the individual.

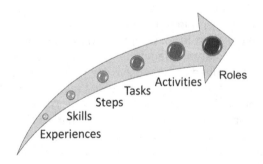

Figure 7.1 Role development according to the Model of Human Occupation showing six (6) dimensions of Doing.
(*Source: adapted from the six dimensions of participation* [de las Heras de Pablo et al. 2017a, 2017b]).

Box 7.5   Author's note

by Sue Parkinson

Learning about the Model of Human Occupation (Kielhofner 2005) was a revelation to me. In retrospect, many of my student placements had led me to focus on occupational performance in terms of a person's safety or independence. If a person was able to complete everyday tasks safely and independently in the health setting where they were being assessed, it was assumed that their success would extend to their own homes, despite it being generally acknowledged that the person's environment could impact their performance. I would have felt so much more assured that a person could cope at home if I had been taught to pay attention to their communication and interaction, process skills, and motor skills – the skills that underpin performance in all activities.

MOHO also taught me to articulate the difference between being able to perform a set activity and participating in meaningful occupations over a period of time. Many of the people that I worked with in mental health settings could perform activities perfectly well and yet this ability was not transferred into their everyday lives. The phrase that they used to describe their experience was 'I can, but I don't'. In other words, they could perform the activities if requested to do so, but their ongoing participation was affected by their volition or their habituation.

In summary, Kielhofner's Model of Human Occupation (ed Taylor 2017) does not preclude a focus on occupational performance and neither does it underrate the importance of occupation-based interventions. Indeed, its foremost author stated that

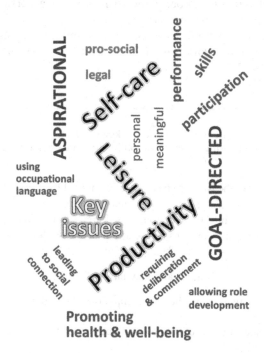

Figure 7.2 Key occupational issues.

occupational therapy's contemporary paradigm reflects three broad themes which clearly reflect the profession's occupational *centre,* its occupational *focus,* and its occupational *base*:

- *'The **centrality** of occupation to health and well-being*
- *Recognition of occupational problems/challenges as the **focus** of therapy*
- *Occupation-**based** practice (use of occupation to improve health status ...'*

(Kielhofner 2009, p49)

So, the Model of Human Occupation recognises the power of occupation-based practice, even though it has earned its reputation as an occupation focused model because of its superb ability to articulate not just *what* people do (the occupational focus), but also *how* occupation is motivated, *how* occupation is organised into patterns of everyday life, and *how* it is performed in the context of the environment. In a complex, dynamic system, MOHO contends that altering any of the following factors can influence what people end up doing:

- the values that are important to them
- the interests that satisfy them
- their obligations and expectations relating to their roles and habits
- their subjective sense of their objective capacity
- the social environment that supports them
- the physical environment where they live their lives

This understanding is crucial when identifying the occupational issues that a person faces. It enables the occupational therapist to personalise the issues so that a work-related issue might be 'achieving work satisfaction' (emphasising volition), 'managing work and home-life' (habituation), 'completing work tasks' (performance), or 'accessing the workplace' (environment) (See Table 7.2).

Table 7.2 Top tips for Key Issues

- When describing the occupational focus of therapy, separate the key issues
- List three or four occupational issues – regarding experiences, skills, steps, tasks, activities, or roles

  o Three is 'the magic number' – it allows the issues to be easily remembered by everyone, so that you can quickly review the person's progress every time you meet. Paradoxically, condensing all the issues into three or four broad areas reduces the possibility of accidentally overlooking any concerns as therapy progresses (Prior and Duncan 2009)

  o The issues should encompass all the person's needs and may have a broad focus

    ▪ If the person only faces one or two issues, then an occupational formulation is unlikely to be needed
    ▪ If the person has multiple issues, then you will need to group them together to form three or four broader issues

(Continued)

Table 7.2 (Continued)

  - The resulting goals should be legal, but do not worry at this point as to whether they are realistic (see how to make goals achievable in Chapter 9)

- Think carefully about how to word the issues

  o The wording should capture the person's motivation and be pitched to match their understanding
  o Each issue should be described in a short phrase (which can then be used in successive goals)
  o Write the issues so that the focus is on occupational change rather than psychological change, e.g., 'gaining paid employment' *rather than* 'having the confidence to apply for jobs'
  o Write the issues using the same language that you use when talking with the person, which might be 'gaining paid employment', but could also be 'getting a job' or 'finding work'. This helps to personalise the issues
  o Write the issues neutrally, rather than describing the problem, e.g., 'gaining paid employment' *not* 'unemployment'. This keeps an upbeat, hopeful mood
  o Do not write the issues as aims at this stage, e.g., write 'gaining paid employment' *not* 'to gain paid employment', as it is important to agree on the issues before placing any expectations on the person

- Think carefully before leaving out any important issues, even if the person worries that they cannot be resolved

  o Reassure the person that you will support them to work towards the goals step by step, and agree all timescales so that they are realistic
  o If necessary, document that the person does not agree with the issue being the focus of therapy, but set a goal so that you can measure whether you are making a difference, and provide positive feedback as the person begins to make progress
  o Consider including a strength that the person can build on, in order to retain a positive focus and to ease the inclusion of more difficult issues

References

Blair SEE (2000) The centrality of occupation during life transitions. *British Journal of Occupational Therapy*, 63(5), 231–237.

Brown T, Bourke-Taylor H (2012) Infusing user-friendly occupational terminology into our daily dialogues and conversations. *British Journal of Occupational Therapy*, 75(11), 48.

Canadian Association of Occupational Therapists [CAOT] (2017). CAOT position statement: occupations and health. *Occupational Now*, 11(1), 24.

Christiansen C, Baum C, Bass-Haugen J, eds. (2005) *Occupational Therapy: Performance, Participation and Well-being,* 3rd ed. Thorofare, NJ: Slack Incorporated.

de las Heras CG, Llerana V, Kielhofner G [posthumous] (2019) *The Remotivation Process: Progressive intervention for individuals with severe volitional challenges: a user's manual. Version 2.0.* Chicago: University of Illinois at Chicago.

de las Heras de Pablo C, Fan C-W, Kielhofner G [posthumous] (2017a) Dimensions of Doing. In RR Taylor, ed. *Kielhofner's Model of Human Occupation: Theory and Application.* Philadelphia: Wolters Kluwer. 107–122.

de las Heras de Pablo C, Parkinson S, Pépin G, Kielhofner G [posthumous] (2017b) Intervention process: enabling occupational change. In RR Taylor, ed. *Kielhofner's Model of Human Occupation: Theory and Application*. Philadelphia: Wolters Kluwer. 195–216.

Di Tommaso A, Isbel S, Scarvell J, Wicks A (2016) Occupational therapists' perceptions of occupation in practice: An exploratory study. *Australian Occupational Therapy Journal, 63(3)*, 206–213.

Fisher AG (2013) Occupation-centred, occupation-based, occupation-focused: same, same or different? *Scandinavian Journal of Occupational Therapy, 20(3)*, 162–173.

Gillen A, Greber C (2014) Occupation-focused practice: challenges and choices *British Journal of Occupational Therapy, 77(1)*, 39–41.

Golledge J (1998) Distinguishing between occupation, purposeful activity and activity, part 1: review and explanation. *British Journal of Occupational Therapy, 61(3)*, 100–105.

Gray JM (1997). Application of the phenomenological method to the concept of occupation. *Journal of Occupational Science, 4(1)*, 5–17.

Gray JM (1998) Putting Occupation into practice: occupation as ends, occupation as means. *American Journal of occupational Therapy, 52(5)*, 354–364.

Greber C (2018) Postmodernism and beyond in occupational therapy. *Australian Occupational Therapy Journal, 65(1)*, 69–72.

Gustafsson L, Molineux M, Bennett S (2014) Contemporary occupational therapy practice: the challenges of being evidence based and philosophically congruent. *Australian Occupational Therapy Journal, 61(2)*, 121–123.

Ilott I, Mounter C (2000) Occupational science: an impossible dream or an agenda for action? *British Journal of Occupational Therapy, 63(5)*, 238–240.

Jackson J, Carlson M, Mandel D, Zemke R, Clark F (1998) Occupation in lifestyle redesign: the Well Elderly Study Occupational Therapy Program. *American Journal of Occupational Therapy, 52(5)*, 326–336.

Joosten AV (2015), Contemporary occupational therapy: our occupational therapy models are essential to occupation centred practice. *Australian Occupational Therapy Journal, 62(3)*, 219–222.

Keponen R, Launiainen H (2008) Using the Model of Human Occupation to nurture an occupational focus in the clinical reasoning of experienced therapists. *Occupational Therapy in Health Care, 22(2-3)*, 95–104.

Kielhofner G (1992) *Conceptual Foundations of Occupational Therapy*. Philadelphia: F.A. Davis.

Kielhofner G (2005) *Model of Human Occupation: Theory and Application*, 3rd ed. Baltimore: Lippincott, Williams & Wilkins.

Kielhofner G (2008) *Model of Human Occupation: Theory and Application*, 4th ed. Baltimore: Lippincott, Williams & Wilkins.

Kielhofner G (2009) *Conceptual Foundations of Occupational Therapy*. 4th ed. FA Davis Company, Philadelphia

Law M Steinwender S, Leclair L (1998) Occupation, health and well-being. *Canadian Journal of Occupational Therapy, 65(2)*, 81–91.

Leclair LL (2010) Re-examining concepts of occupation and occupation-based models: Occupational Therapy and community development. *Canadian Journal of Occupational Therapy, 77(1)*, 15–21.

Mackey H, Nancarrow S (2006) *Enabling Independence: a Guide for Rehabilitation Workers*. Oxford: Blackwell Publishing.

Mattingly C (1994) Clinical revision: changing the therapeutic story in midstream. In: C Mattingly, MH Fleming eds. *Clinical Reasoning: Forms of Inquiry in a Therapeutic Practice*. Philadelphia: F.A. Davis Company. 270–291.

Pereira RB (2015) Occupare, to seize: expanding the potential of occupation in contemporary practice. *Australian Occupational Therapy Journal, 62(3)*, 208–209.

Pettican A, Bryant W (2007) Sustaining a focus on occupation in Community Mental Health practice. *British Journal of Occupational Therapy, 70(4)*, 140–146.

Pierre BL (2001) Occupational Therapy as documented in patients records Part III. Valued but not documented: underground practice in the context of professional written communication, *Scandinavian Journal of Occupational Therapy, 8(4)*, 174–183.

Poulden D, Oke LE (1990) Occupational therapy in Australia — where are we going and how do we get there? *Australian Occupational Therapy Journal, 37(3)*, 147–149.

Prior S, Duncan EAS (2009) Assessment skills for practice. In: Duncan EAS, ed. *Skills for Practice in Occupational Therapy.* Churchill Livingstone. 75–90.

Taylor RR ed. (2017) *Kielhofner's Model of Human Occupation.* 5th ed. Philadelphia: Wolters Kluwer.

Taylor RR, Kielhofner G [posthumous] (2017) Introduction to the Model of Human Occupation. In: RR Taylor ed. *Kielhofner's Model of Human Occupation.* 5th ed. Philadelphia: Wolters Kluwer. 3–10.

Townsend E, Wilcock A (2004) Occupational justice. In: CH Christiansen, EA Townsend eds. *Introduction to Occupation, the Art and Science of Living.* Upper Saddle River, NJ: Prentice Hall. 243–273.

Turner A, Alsop A (2015) Unique core skills: exploring occupational therapists' hidden assets. *British Journal of Occupational Therapy, 78(12)*, 739–749.

Twinley R (2013) The dark side of occupation: a concept for consideration. *Australian Occupational Therapy Journal, 60(4)*, 301–303.

Whiteford G, Townsend E, Hocking C (2000) Reflections on the renaissance of occupation. *Canadian Journal of Occupational Therapy, 67(1)*, 61–69.

Wilcock AA (2006) *An Occupational Perspective of Health.* 2nd ed. Thorofare, NJ: Slack.

Wilcock A, Townsend E (2000) Occupational terminology interactive dialogue: occupational justice. *Journal of Occupational Science: Australia, 7(2)*, 84–86.

World Federation of Occupational Therapists [WFOT] (2012) Definition of occupational therapy. Available at: https://www.facebook.com/thewfot/posts/definition-of-occupational-therapyat-the-2012-council-meeting-it-was-agreed-to-r/360545177371670/ Accessed 31/07/2019.

8 Wrapping up the formulation

Occupational therapists are required to record a 'justifiable account' or a 'rationale' for all that they do (Royal College of Occupational Therapists [RCOT] 2018) and yet occupational therapy records sometimes fail to document professional reasoning or link interventions to goals (*ibid*). A well-crafted occupational formulation remedies this situation by recording the therapist's decision-making while taking into account an individual's preferences and choices. Its intention is to be as comprehensible as possible so that all those involved can understand how the decisions have been made, while still meeting all legal obligations regarding documentation. In order for this to be accomplished, the main content of a formulation benefits from

- being prefaced by a brief introduction detailing the circumstances in which the formulation has been made and clearly identifying the individual concerned
- and by ending with a concise summary of the main factors affecting the person's identity and competence

Introduction

Clark and Youngstrom (2013) described the suggested content for screening reports and their recommendations could easily be applied to all occupational formulation structures. Although the content is not organised in the same way, it is suggested that screening reports should include a person's occupational history (their pattern of occupation, values, interests, and goals), an occupational profile (their strengths and limitations), and any recommendations regarding the need for occupational therapy. These elements all fit neatly into the three main sections of an occupational formulation. However, Clark and Youngstrom also recommend that screening reports should include

- personal identification details
- referral information
- a record of assessments that have been used

This essential information can be included in a formulation's introduction.

Personal identification details

Clark and Youngstrom recommend that all rrts should start with listing personal details for the purpose of identification, such as the person's name, date of birth, and gender. To

DOI: 10.4324/9781003046301-8

this one might add the person's preferred name and their known address or other demographic information regarding the person's marital status or ethnicity. One may also be required to include a unique identifier or code to assist in the delivery of safe integrated care (RCOT 2018), as well as the person's health status and applicable diagnoses, and any significant precautions or contraindications (Clark and Youngstrom 2013).

The inclusion of a person's diagnosis may not be essential to an occupational formulation, as occupational therapy differs from the medical model in many respects (Yerxa 1991), and diagnosis alone is an insufficient guide for occupational therapy (Rogers 1982, Macneil et al. 2012, Thompson 2012). Yet even though medical diagnosis does not predict function (Lollar and Simeonsson 2005), it may 'conjure up certain images' relating to a person's occupational status (Rogers and Holm 1991), and it is the occupational therapist's task to consider how a diagnostic condition might influence how a person functions (Fleming 1991). Therefore, occupational therapists should have an understanding of the processes and prognoses of their clients' health conditions, and recognise when they are drawing on related knowledge from the medical model (Kielhofner 2004).

Referral information

Referral information may include the date and source of referral and the services requested or the reason for referral (Clark and Youngstrom 2013). This may be required for the purposes of various referral prioritisation policies (Harries and Gilhooly 2003), or may be used to audit whether referrals to occupational therapy are appropriate, or may support research studying links between initial referrals and eventual goals. Furthermore, therapists may need to make a case, or rather *formulate* a case, for working with an individual for entirely different reasons than those stated on referral. Only by placing the formulation in the context of the original referral can therapists begin to educate those involved in the person's care regarding their profession's true potential.

Occupational assessments

Records need to be comprehensive and therapists must be able to demonstrate that their interventions are based on sound assessment (RCOT 2018). However, individual assessments will already have been recorded in detail and so there is no need to replicate or restate the findings in a formulation's introduction. Rather, the formulation needs to be linked to the assessments, and a brief list of completed assessments is all that is required at this point.

The most important consideration for including an assessment is that it should be occupational or profession-specific. Profession-specific assessments reflect the profession's particular responsibility (Haglund and Henriksson 2003), and quickly establish a clinician's credentials for constructing an occupational formulation. It is also recommended that evidence-based measures should be included (College of Occupational Therapists [COT] 2013), although non-standardised assessment methods are valid sources of information (Hinojosa et al. 2010) and may be included in the list (see Table 8.1).

Box 8.1   Author's note

by Dr Rob Brooks

The main thing to remember when writing the introduction is that this is not where the story starts. The real story begins in the Identity section, where everything that is of significance to the person is captured. You could say, that the introduction includes the boring information – the information that is already generally known – so do not make it even more boring by writing too much. Enough said!

Table 8.1 Top tips for the Introduction

- Keep brief – all the information has already been documented elsewhere in the person's notes
- Do not include any occupational information here, even if this came with the referral (e.g., regarding the person's social history, where they live, or how many children they have)

  o All occupational information needs to be integrated into either the Identity or Competence section with as little duplication as possible
  o If you include occupational information in the introduction you may forget to refer to it in the main body of the formulation and miss key issues

- Save yourself time by ordering the information systematically and following the same order every time e.g.,

  o Name, age, and gender
  o Diagnosis or health conditions (including physical and mental health concerns)
  o Reason for referral to (or contact with) Occupational Therapy
  o Occupational assessments completed

- Write names of evidence-based assessments in full, and include a brief reference if they are standardised, to show that the formulation is based on sound reasoning

Summary

The process of writing an elegant formulation resembles the artistic creation of a short story, with a beginning (the person's identity), a middle (the person's competence), and an end (the occupational focus). Yet formulations also need to function as formal means of communication with elements that have more in common with scientific evaluations. Although they exist for the benefit of an individual rather than the general public, formulations need to bear all the hallmarks of good health communication as defined by Bernhardt (2004):

'Health communication is the scientific development, strategic dissemination, and critical evaluation of relevant, accessible, and understandable health information communicated to and from intended audiences to advance the health of the public' (p2051)

As a formal means of communication, occupational formulations begin with an introduction that confirms the person's name, age, and gender, and sets the formulation within the context of healthcare provision. They also benefit from having concise summaries that provide the readers with a précis of the findings. These help to optimise the communication in an efficient manner while still demonstrating empathy for the needs of the person (Schiavo 2013), by summarising the 'nature, balance, pattern, and context of occupations and activities' (Creek 2003, p8) in the person's life.

Elevator speech

Given the sheer volume of evidence that needs to be sifted through in healthcare settings (Peek 2003), it is inevitable that some readers will skim through reports to reach the conclusion. For this reason, the intention of the summary is not to introduce new information, but to pique the readers' interest (Monty 2014). By encouraging readers to read the back story, the summary also provides the therapist with a prepared 'elevator speech' to hook people's interest in face-to-face conversations. An elevator speech is a business expression that refers to a short persuasive speech (Simpson 2016) which makes the most of incidental encounters. Although not essential for successful communication, it can help the speaker to make connections and invite further conversations (Denning and Dew 2012). In today's fast-paced world, it is arguably incumbent upon all professionals to be able to give clear and concise summaries of their work (Simpson 2016). At the very least, this should help to avoid the embarrassment of failing to find the right words at the right time (MacLean 2012), but more than this it may help to reduce the type of suboptimal communication that is all too often associated with untoward events (Haig et al. 2006).

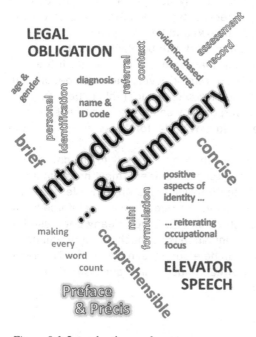

Figure 8.1 Introduction and summary.

Formulation in miniature

Jacobs (2012) considers that occupational therapists cannot assume their beliefs will be known or shared by their readers, and urges her fellow therapists to use words skilfully. She declares that,

> *'Occupational therapy practitioners only become accomplished communicators when they can effectively communicate that occupation is essential to individuals' and society's health and well-being. We are health communicators and the words we use are important'* (p653)

This means that a summary must be 'compelling to the target audience ... instructive ... easy to understand and to remember" (*ibid,* p669) – a formulation in miniature.

Drafting the summary forces occupational therapists to think about the words they use and make every word count (see Table 8.2) so that they can be ready with a short meaningful answer to the question 'how can occupational therapy help this person?' By advocating for the occupational needs of their clients as clearly and concisely as possible, they maximise their chances of being rewarded by durable multi-disciplinary collaborations working towards a common end (Peek 2003). Indeed, not only will they have a ready-made elevator speech when time is scarce, they will be more likely to *elevate* and engage their listener's understanding in the time that is available (Jones 2015).

Box 8.2   Author's note

by Sue Parkinson

   When my colleagues and I were first learning to write summary statements, the temptation to try to include all the preceding information in the formulation proved to be irresistible to some. This not only destroyed the whole point of writing the summary, but also took up precious time. Eventually, I came up with the top tips for writing a summary (see below) and I advise you to follow these.

   I think that it is particularly important to start with positives from the Identity section, as this may be the only section that team members read. If the only purpose served by the summary is to remind everyone that people are individuals with strengths to build on then I would consider this to be a massive achievement. In fact, it serves a dual purpose, by sending a clear message that occupational therapists are prepared to advocate for those they have the privilege of working with.

   The second part of the summary can then be devoted to describing the issues that affect the person's competence. Readers may have scanned through the issues that occupational therapy will focus on, but referring back to the issues in the summary provides a valuable opportunity to reinforce them. In fact, I recommend reusing the exact words that have already been used to define the issues, because good communication is as much about repetition as it is about being articulate, and there can be eloquence in simplicity. The same words will also be used at the heart of each successive goal, so this is your chance to fix the words in your memory.

Table 8.2 Top tips for the summary

- Ensure that the summary is between 80 and 120 words long. Any fewer and you will not do justice to the person's story. Any more and you risk making the information too difficult to recall
- Do not include any new information
- Start with one or two sentences that are wholly positive about the person's identity

    o List key roles and interests

- End by reiterating and contextualising the key issues

    o Reiterate the key by using the same words that have already been used to define them
    o Put each issue in context, either by including a little piece of information from the identity section regarding the person's motivation or a small piece of information from the competence section regarding specific strengths or limitations, barriers, or supports
    o Cultivate an optimistic style of writing – If the person is keen to work towards future goals this is easy enough to do. If they a pessimistic about whether any of the issues can be resolved, there is no need to refer to their doubts in the summary. Instead, you can reiterate the issues in the form of recommendations, indicating that the person would benefit from addressing the issues

---

References

Bernhardt JM (2004) Communication at the core of effective public health. *American Journal of Public Health, 94(12)*, 2051–2053.

Clark GF, Youngstrom MJ (2013) Guidelines for documentation of Occupational Therapy. *American Journal of Occupational Therapy, 67(6)*, S32–S38.

College of Occupational Therapists [COT] (2013) *Position Statement: Occupational Therapists' Use of Standardised Outcome Measures*. London: COT

Creek J (2003) *Occupational Therapy Defined as a Complex Intervention*. London: College of Occupational Therapists.

Denning PJ, Dew N (2012) The profession of IT: the myth of the elevator pitch. *Communications of the Association for Computing Machinery, 55(6)*, 38–40.

Fleming MH (1991) Clinical reasoning in medicine compared with clinical reasoning in occupational therapy. *American Journal of Occupational Therapy, 45(11)*, 988–996.

Haglund L, HenrikssonC (2003). Concepts in occupational therapy in relation to the ICF. *Occupational Therapy International, 10*, 253–268.

Haig KM, Sutton S, Whittington J (2006) SBAR: a shared mental model for improving communication between clinicians. *Journal of Quality and Patient Safety, 32(3)*, 167–175.

Harries P, Gilhooly K (2003) Identifying occupational therapists' referral priorities in community health. *Occupational Therapy International, 10(2)*, 150–164.

Hinojosa J, Kramer P, Crist (2010). *Evaluation: Obtaining and Interpreting Data*. 3rd ed. Bethesda, MD: AOTA Press.

Jacobs, K. (2012) PromOTing occupational therapy: words, images, and actions (Eleanor Clarke Slagle Lecture). *American Journal of Occupational Therapy, 66(6)*, 652–671.

Jones L (2015) Using your Occupational Therapy "Elevator Speech" to effectively ELEVATE understanding of the profession! Gotta Be OT blog. https://gottabeot.wordpress.com/2015/01/27/using-your-occupational-therapy-elevator-speech-to-effectively-elevate-understanding-of-the-profession/. Accessed 08/08/2019.

Kielhofner G (2004) *Conceptual Foundations of Occupational Therapy*. 3rd ed. Philadelphia: FA Davis Co.

Lollar DJ, Simeonsson RJ (2005) Diagnosis to function: classification for children and youths. *Journal of Developmental & Behavioral Pediatrics, 26(4),* 323–330.

MacLean R (2012) The elevator pitch. *Environmental Quality Management, 21(4),* 99–105.

Macneil CA, Hasty MK, Conus P, Berk M (2012) Is diagnosis enough to guide interventions in mental health? Using case formulation in clinical practice. *BMC Medicine, 10,* 111. DOI: 10. 1186/1741-7015-10-111. Accessed 08/08/2019.

Monty DA (2014) *Sales Hunting: How to Develop New Territories and Major Accounts in Half the Time Using Trust As Your Weapon.* Berkley CA: Apress, Berkeley.

Peek, C J (2003) An Evidence-based "Elevator Speech" for a practical world: Comment. *Families, Systems, & Health, 21(2),* 135–139.

Royal College of Occupational Therapists [RCOT] (2018) *Keeping Records: Guidance For Occupational Therapists.* London: RCOT

Rogers JC (1982) Order and disorder in Occupational Therapy. *American Journal of Occupational Therapy, 36(1),* 29–35.

Rogers JC, Holm MB (1991) Occupational therapy diagnostic reasoning: a component of clinical reasoning. *American Journal of Occupational Therapy, 45(11),* 1045–1053.

Schiavo R (2013) *Health Communication: From Theory to Practice,* 2nd ed. San Francisco: Jossey-Bass.

Simpson D (2016) "Going up?" A sport psychology consultant's guide to the elevator speech. *Journal of Sport Psychology in Action, 7(2),* 109–120.

Thompson BF (2012) Abductive reasoning and case formulation in complex cases. In: L Robertson ed. *Clinical Reasoning in Occupational Therapy.* Pondicherry: Wiley-Blackwell. 15–30.

Yerxa EJ (1991) Seeking a relevant, ethical and realistic way of knowing Occupational Therapy. *American Journal of Occupational Therapy, 45(3),* 199–204.

9 Negotiating measurable occupational goals

Expectations

Goal setting is thought to be an essential step in the therapeutic process (Page et al. 2015), or if not essential, then certainly indicative of best practice (Waller 2015), and something that is increasingly expected of occupational therapists (World Federation of Occupational Therapists et al. 2019). Indeed, goal setting has become a legislative requirement (Levack et al. 2006a) and is even practised in palliative care (Boa et al. 2014) where, despite limited time and potential, it may serve to affirm the value of the life that an individual still has left to enjoy (Duncan 2016). There is also evidence that it is practised across the breadth of rehabilitation services, including neurological, medical, and mental health care (Levack et al. 2015) and its role has been summed up as follows,

> 'Goal setting is considered an essential part of clinical rehabilitation. It has been described as a core practice within rehabilitation, a requirement for effective interdisciplinary teamwork, and an activity that specifically characterises both rehabilitation services and those who provide them. In clinical practice, there has been a growing emphasis on the need for interventions to be goal-oriented. Goal terminology is becoming integral to discussions of guidelines, policies and professional requirements'

(Levack et al. 2015, p8)

The strongest case for goal setting relates to its impact on the process of therapy. Goals are thought to enable individuals to plan for the future, which generates a sense of hope, and increases their motivation and persistence towards goal attainment (Waller 2015). Also, when goals have been negotiated with all those concerned, they have been linked to an increased sense of ownership and strengthened motivation to engage in therapy (Armstrong 2008), as the individuals are better able to understand the purpose of interventions (Page et al. 2015). Thereafter, greater engagement in therapy is associated with positive outcomes (Brewer et al. 2014) and may even lead to individuals being more able and likely to set their own goals in the future (Annesi 2002).

Goal setting certainly seems to bestow advantages to therapists by allowing them to hone their professional reasoning – or their understanding of the challenges faced by their clients (Paterson and Summerfield-Mann 2006) – and so communicate the focus of therapy (Waller 2015). This focus can be shared with the individual, with relatives and carers, with the wider team and with those funding the service, and can confer a clearer sense of direction for all stakeholders (Page et al. 2015). In turn, this should produce

DOI: 10.4324/9781003046301-9

more individualised care and better quality feedback (Law et al. 2004, Park 2009), more effective use of time and resources (Park 2009), and improved continuity of care (Scott and Haggerty 1984). Any time spent in identifying goals at the outset is thought to be saved later, not only because interventions are more meaningful and targeted, but because conflict within the team is reduced and multidisciplinary collaboration is improved (Armstrong 2008).

There are numerous reports of improved outcomes being attributed to goal setting (Scott and Haggerty 1984, Annesi 2002, Arnetz et al. 2004). It has been associated with increased quality of life (Waller 2015) and is valued as an effective mechanism for enhancing self-management strategies (Garvey et al. 2015). Evidence regarding its effectiveness is developing, particularly in child therapy services where positive impacts on goal attainment have been noted (Scobbie et al. 2013), and positive care outcomes have been attributed to services focused on working towards outcomes that meet the needs of children and their families (Kolehmainen et al. 2012). In one particular study, the efficacy of two different goal-setting approaches was investigated (Vroland-Nordstrand et al. 2016): in one, the goals were self-identified by the children; and in the other, the goals were identified by the parents. Both approaches yielded increases in mean goal attainment, which were sustained after 5 months, and both were equally effective. It is perhaps even more intriguing to learn that client-identified goals have been found to be just as effective in an adult group that proceeded to receive an intervention, compared with a control group that received no intervention (Herdman et al. 2018). This suggests that goal-setting might be regarded as an intervention in its own right.

Box 9.1   Author's note

by Sue Parkinson

I would be less fervent about the value of measurable goals if I had not witnessed their impact on practice. Once my colleagues and I had mastered the art of writing measurable goals, we checked how our work was perceived by others (Parkinson et al. 2011) and were buoyed up by the comments we received.

- *service users* spoke about how the goals had been instrumental in helping them to work towards so many of their long-held aspirations, and also how having goals had helped them to restart activities that they had stopped. They described 'getting back to work', 'finding voluntary work', 'going back to the gym', as well as 'developing new interests', and 'following new routines'. The goals helped them to 'stay focussed and keep up the momentum', and it was acknowledged that 'I needed someone to give me that extra nudge', and 'the OT has helped me to clarify what I need and how to go about it'
- a *carer* described how a relative was 'looking forward to being able to do things on his own and becoming more self-confident' because he had goals to work towards
- *support workers* also noted that the people they worked with had responded well to having clear goals. The goals gave them something to focus on and enabled them to recognise the progress that they were making, but the difference seemed

to be more fundamental in that the goals gave people hope and even allowed individuals to develop a more positive view of themselves.

- *social workers* echoed the views of support workers when they said that the goals enabled them to stay on track by providing 'a clearly planned timeframe'
- a *nurse* voiced her opinion that the goals 'helped us to link very effectively with the occupational therapy department'
- *occupational therapists* were both relieved and proud when they discovered that the structure of the goals made them 'easy to communicate and share with others', thereby allowing other professions to recognise the unique contribution of Occupational Therapy

Limitations

Despite the theoretical benefits of goal setting being well-documented (Parkinson et al. 2011), a note of caution is still advisable. Although an increasing amount of research is being conducted (Levack et al. 2015), much of the research has not been of the highest quality (Duncan 2016). Moreover, systematic reviews of randomised controlled trials have concluded that evidence regarding the impact of goal setting on clinical outcomes is inconsistent at best (Levack et al. 2015), and inconclusive or poor at worst (Levack et al. 2016).

The problem appears to stem from the fact that goal setting is a complex skill (Bowman et al. 2015), and approaches to goal–setting vary with no consensus regarding the best approach (Levack et al. 2016), and a high level of variability in goal-setting practice (Scobbie et al. 2014). Guidelines may be present, but a standardised method of writing and evaluating goals does not exist (Bowman et al. 2015). Moreover, therapists may be unsure about how to implement client-centred practice (Armstrong 2008) and the situation becomes more difficult when their clients are dealing with the prospect of diminishing abilities (Boa et al. 2014) or have limited capacity. Occupational therapists have the added challenge of trying to write occupation-focused goals in services where medical models still predominate. This was thought to be a factor influencing the results of an analysis undertaken of 335 occupational therapy plans, in which it was found that there were no occupational goals in 42% of them (Page et al. 2015). In addition, 45% of the goals were not regarded as being specific, 33% were deemed unrealistic, and 59% were not considered to be measurable.

Even when specific goals are attempted, it seems that therapists rarely use these goals to allocate available resources, and rarely evaluate the effects of their treatments (Kolehmainen et al. 2012). Furthermore, when goals are evaluated positively, there may still be unintended consequences if the biggest issues have been prioritised to the detriment of smaller everyday issues (Duncan 2016). In addition to these concerns, there are fundamental difficulties in evaluating goal attainment itself. For instance, Goal Attainment Scaling (GAS) (Kiresuk and Sherman 1968) has grown in popularity in occupational therapy but is acknowledged to have limitations (Weidenbohm et al. 2005). It has also been criticised for not being able to discriminate between (a) the outcomes of substandard therapy oriented toward easily achievable goals, and (b) therapy of a higher standard where ambitious goals are achieved (Levack 2018).

Of course, it could be argued that if one of the most important reasons for goal setting is to motivate the individual, then a sense of personal achievement is more important than goal attainment at a service level. For this reason, albeit that goal setting might be viewed as an alien concept by individuals who are unused to planning for the future (Kielhofner and Barrett 1998), it is disappointing to note that goals are not always shared with the very people for whom they are intended. In a study of goal setting in children's services, it was found that therapists rarely shared goals with either the child or the parents (Kolehmainen et al. 2012), and in another study in acute inpatient services, it was discovered that the majority of service users and carers felt that they had not been genuinely involved in planning their treatment (Simpson et al. 2017). Some said that their views had not been listened to - an occurrence which was mirrored in a third study showing that therapists tended to focus on goals that could be achieved within a residential setting, relating to 'programming and symptom management' despite the residents wanting to prioritise community involvement (Richard and Knis-Matthews 2010). In yet another study (Saito et al. 2019), it was found that there was a match between only 21% of goals reported by occupational therapists and their rehabilitation clients, even when both perceived that they had engaged in goal-setting together.

Box 9.2   Author's note

by Sue Parkinson

Despite all the limitations of goal-setting, I believe that it is worth persisting, not just because of the positive feedback given by those involved (see previous Author's note). Goal-setting is certainly a complex skill, but I believe it can be made easier when underpinned by a robust formulation. In addition, I aim to share a standardised method for writing goals rather than merely describing their desired qualities.

I cannot claim that my own attempt to audit goal-attainment was of the highest quality, given the logistical constraints of gathering data in a service with limited resources. It was never published, but I continue to be encouraged by its results as it indicated that the majority of goals being negotiated in a county-wide UK occupational therapy service could be attained. Goals were either all met or almost all met in 66.5% of cases. As might be expected, fewer goals were met within the time available in our adult acute mental health services (where 43% of goals were either 'all met' or 'almost all met'), but figures were higher in adult community mental health services (70%), child and adolescent mental health services (73%), adult rehabilitation services and older adult acute services (both 75%), and older adult community services (84%).

Good practice

Goal setting is just a stage in a treatment process and successful goal setting is, therefore, dependent on the stages that come before it. This starts with gathering the perspectives of all concerned during the assessment phase (Kolehmainen et al. 2013). It is at this point that occupational therapists often choose an occupational model to support their goal planning, and while there are a number of occupational models and assessments that could be used, the Model of Human Occupation (ed. Taylor 2017) is certainly the most developed model in terms of practical resources, with around 20 varied assessments that complement each other (Wong and Fisher 2015). All models, however, are regarded as having the potential to raise occupational therapy practice from the mere application of techniques to a professional process which blends conceptual problem solving, planning, and action' (Kielhofner 2009, Joosten 2015). It has even been asserted, that occupational therapists who fail to draw on their occupational models, risk not knowing what their clients want, need, or are expected to do (Joosten 2015).

When goal setting commences, it starts with listening to a person's aspirations (McPherson et al. 2014) and discovering what is meaningful to the person (Dekker et al. 2020), and progresses to identifying clear, specific, and meaningful goals, agreeing on these goals with all parties, and evaluating the progress made thereafter (Kolehmainen et al. 2012). This requires that goals are negotiated (Scobbie et al. 2013, 2014), that roles and responsibilities are agreed in advance, and comparisons between the baseline, current, and target levels are made when reviewing progress (Kolehmainen et al. 2013). Finally, occupational therapists must provide feedback and move on to the next round of decision-making (Scobbie et al. 2013, 2014). These processes should be emphasised throughout an occupational therapist's training, as evidence exists that training can enhance both goal setting and client participation (Flink et al. 2016). Moreover, therapists can continue to develop their goal-setting skills by adopting standardised methods of writing and evaluating goals (Bowman et al. 2015).

Whatever else therapists might do, it is universally considered to be good practice to enter into a partnership in which therapy is more about collaboration and facilitation than direction or imposition (Armstrong 2008). This undoubtedly requires skills and effort (*ibid*) to ensure that rapport is built, the person's concerns are listened to, their priorities are incorporated, workable solutions are identified through a process of joint problem-solving, goals are defined using accessible language, and the person is involved in monitoring progress at all stages (Tang Yan et al. 2014, Waller 2015). Naturally, this is easier with some people than others (Randall and McEwan 2000) as not all service users want to participate in shared decision-making (Park 2009) or have the capacity to do so (Doig et al. 2009). However, it should be recognised that only a minimal level of medical/psychiatric stability is required to negotiate meaningful goals (Linhorst et al. 2002) and the extra time that needs to be set aside (Park 2009) can be saved later (Armstrong 2008). Collaboration is therefore deemed to be worth the investment of time, energy, and resources (Brewer et al. 2014), including necessary education and supervision (Armstrong 2008). It is an integral part of the therapy process (Brewer et al. 2014) which facilitates participation and enhances goal-directed rehabilitation (Doig et al. 2009). Indeed, the importance of occupational therapists working in partnership with the people they serve is supported by,

> '*Evidence that greater involvement of service users in decisions about their interventions improves health outcomes, satisfaction with services and reduces costs*'
> (College of Occupational Therapists [COT] 2013, p1)

Box 9.3   Author's note
by Dr Rob Brooks
The process of negotiating goals becomes so much smoother when the key issues have been already agreed during the formulation process, and when the

therapist follows a clear method for writing goals. Even in those cases, when people may appreciate general aims but not see the need for writing specific goals, you may be able to win them over in time. Initially, it may be all that you can do, to let them know that *you* need to set goals so that you can measure whether your interventions have made a difference. As time goes by, however, when you are able to provide them with specific feedback about their progress, they may be inclined to collaborate more fully in the process of negotiation.

How smart is SMART?

The acronym that is frequently used to guide goal–setting is SMART (Bovend'Eerdt et al. 2009), and many therapists will have an understanding of the qualities represented by the letters S, M, A, R, and T. Interestingly, these initials have been interpreted differently over time, and there is no consensus regarding its best interpretation (Levack et al. 2015). It is commonly understood to mean that goals should be *Specific, Measurable, Achievable, Realistic, and Timed* (Waller 2015), however, S might also be interpreted as being succinct (McPherson et al. 2014), A has also been interpreted as *Agreed* (Page et al. 2015) or Aspirational (McPherson et al. 2014), R might also refer to being *Relevant* (Levack et al. 2015), and T could mean Transparent (McPherson et al. 2014). Other acronyms have also been suggested), such as COAST (Gateley and Borcherding 2012) and RUMBA (Barnett 1999) – see below – but it seems as though none of them lead to a standardised method of writing goals (Bowman et al. 2015).

C – Client – who will achieve the goal?	R – Relevant
O – Occupation – focused on which occupation?	U – Understandable
A – Assist level – with what level of assistance/independence?	M – Measurable
S – Specific condition – under what conditions?	B – Behavioural
T – Timeline – by when?	A – Achievable

Specific

A critical appraisal by Mary Law et al. (2004) found that goal attainment is improved when the goals are specific. But which components should be specific? Many assume that goals should specify an element of performance – an action – so that the goals might include the phrase that the person 'is able to do' certain activities (College of Occupational Therapists [COT] 2016), whether these are activities of daily living (ADL) or instrumental activities of daily living (IADL) – activities required in order to participate in self-care, productivity, or leisure. In other words, it means that goals centre on 'goal behaviours (i.e., ADL and IADL tasks) that reflect the values defined by the client' (Schell et al. 2013, p629). Yet observable actions are perhaps better described as being objectives or targets rather than valued goals. Indeed, both the COAST and SMART acronyms have been described as formats for recording 'objectives' (RCOT 2018). Also, the S in COAST stands for 'specific conditions' rather than specific actions, and this is echoed in the College of Occupational Therapists' standards for goal setting (COT 2016) which states that individualised goals require,

'Qualifiers such as level of ability, performance, or participation and any requirement for supervision, assistance, equipment, or adaptation' (p1)

Box 9.4   Author's note
by Sue Parkinson

One of the main recommendations I give when teaching people to write measurable goals is to rethink the meaning of the word 'specific'. If you reduce a person's goals to specific targets or actions – then you risk losing the sense of meaning that their dreams and hopes for the future embody.

Let's take the aim of 'being healthy'. It might be more specific to say that the person should

- lose weight
- go jogging
- learn to relax
- and participate in any number of other activities, such as walking the dog

Now, instead of having one goal, the poor person has at least four activities to remember, and they are likely to encounter all sorts of obstacles on the way. They might not have enough money to participate in some activities or it might be raining when they plan to go jogging, but does this mean that they will automatically fail their overall aim of being healthier?

Another thing that some occupational therapists often try to specify are the exact interventions:

- to attend certain groups
- to complete certain therapies
- to visit certain agencies etc., etc., etc.

However, it is not the person's goal to be a patient, and it is not the person's goal to attend hospital appointments. These interventions are only the means to an end, and should not be confused with the things that are really important to the person.

Let us go back to what the person actually wants – their hopes, their dreams, and try not to tamper with these or to re-word them. Your job is not to limit a person's dreams, but to see how far you can take them on their journey.

So, the first thing you need to do is to *specify* the key occupational words in the three or four issues that are the focus of therapy. Hold on to these keywords. By continuing to re-use the keywords in the goals, it is much more likely that everyone involved in the person's therapy will remember what is important for the person. Instead of changing the keywords and stipulating specific actions or interventions, all you need to do next is to add *specific conditions* to form a goal.

Measurable

Goals need to be measurable so that progress towards the goals can be evaluated (Kolehmainen et al. 2012) and the impact of therapy on goal achievement can be gauged (Waller 2015). Once again, when considering what should be measured, it seems to be the general wisdom that therapists should measure a person's ability to perform a task, so that goals are 'measurable and task-oriented' (Page et al. 2015, p10). Yet progress is a dynamic process that involves 'simultaneous and interactive alterations' (de las Heras de Pablo et al. 2017, p196) which are difficult to pin down to specific actions. The Model of Human Occupation (ed. Taylor 2017) reminds therapists that people must actively participate in developing self-knowledge and that progressive facilitation of volition (motivation for doing) is the basis for goal achievement. So, rather than measuring outward actions, a case can be made for goals being more meaningful when therapists measure the active changes made by the person (Parkinson 2014) which are more inward, meaningful, and sustainable. This can be done by measuring how a person achieves change through a process of occupational engagement (Pépin 2017) in which the person chooses, commits to, explores, identifies, negotiates, plans, practises, re-examines, and ultimately sustains their occupational engagement (Kielhofner and Forsyth 2008).

Box 9.5 Author's note

by Dr Rob Brooks

If a goal has been devised to measure an inner change rather than an external action, one might anticipate that goal attainment would be difficult to measure. Yet, in my experience, measuring objective change is equally challenging because setting a timescale in which a person will be 'able' to do something that they struggle with currently is almost impossible at times. In addition, a therapist might believe that a person has accomplished a task and think that a goal has been attained, and yet the person might think that they did not accomplish the task to their own satisfaction, or with the level of enjoyment that they anticipated.

When measuring an inner change, the therapist is obliged to involve the person, not only in negotiating the goal, but also in measuring their goal attainment. The therapist measures the inner change by asking the person and key others whether they have made a *choice*, what they have discovered in their *exploration*, which pros and cons they have *identified,* what has been *negotiated* or *planned, how much they have practised,* what their *re-examination* has revealed, and whether progress has been *sustained*. The process of evaluation is entirely person-centred.

Box 9.6 Author's note

by Sue Parkinson

I was so excited when I came across the process of engagement in the Model of Human Occupation (Kielhofner and Forsyth 2008, Pépin 2017) and realised that it could be used to measure a person's progress. It provided me with a technique that helped to make a person's long-term goals so much more achievable. After all, I might never know when a person will be able to reach their goal, and at the outset, I might not even know how best to help them, but I can always collaborate with a person to help them to work towards their goals. To do this, it is important to recognise that lasting change does not occur in the therapy sessions, but that time needs to be devoted for a person to assimilate changes, to make adjustments, and ultimately to adapt by

- *choosing* or deciding on a specific way forward might be the first step on the journey
- *committing* to a course of action might be the next step, but beware of using this verb in a goal as it can sound like an order
- *exploring* resources, facilities, and various options might help the person to commit to something
- *identifying* may sound like *choosing*, but in this taxonomy, it means weighing things up by recognising advantages and disadvantages, strengths and limitations, opportunities and constraints
- *negotiating* is an important verb to use if a third party is involved and time needs to be set aside to ensure their agreement
- *planning* might seem like an odd verb to use in a treatment plan – surely the plan has just been written – but it allows for more detailed planning to be developed: who is going to do what, where, when, and how
- *practising* is what occupational therapy is all about. If we say that a person 'will be able to do something', the goal immediately becomes less achievable, because how well the person manages to do something will always be open to interpretation. Stipulating that someone will practise something is much more achievable
- *re-examining* something might happen after a period of practice, or it may occur earlier in the process of change
- *sustaining* is the only verb that means the person will be able to maintain an occupational change, and many occupational therapists actually prefer the verb *maintain* on the basis that this sounds less demanding
- to these verbs, I would add *experiencing* which is the very earliest level of doing, described by de las Heras de Pablo (2011) and her colleagues (2017) (see Figure 7.1 in Chapter 7)

The word 'experience' is also used by Pépin (2017) when she describes how occupational engagement facilitates the process of change. She builds on the work of Kielhofner and Forsyth (2008) and proposes that:

- *exploration* and *practice* help in building *experience*
- that *re-examination* and *negotiation* are needed after this for *interpretation* and *anticipation* (which I associate with *identification and planning*); and
- that a person's eventual *choices* require *commitment* to be *sustained*

A precedent for setting goals that emphasise learning rather than performance can be found in *Learning versus performance goals: When should each be used?* by Seijts and Latham (2005), whose findings are well worth reading.

> '*Setting a specific challenging performance goal has a detrimental effect on a person's effectiveness in the early stages of learning. This is because in the early stage of learning, before effective performance routines have been identified and have become automatic, a person's attention needs to be focused on discovering and mastering the processes required to perform well, rather than on the attainment of a specific level of performance. The attentional demands that can be imposed on people are limited. Trying to attain a specific challenging performance goal places additional demands on people, so much so that they are unable to devote the necessary cognitive resources to mastering the task. A performance outcome goal often distracts attention from the discovery of task-relevant strategies. For example, focusing on a golf score of 95 by novices may prevent them from focusing on the mastery of the swing and weight transfer and using the proper clubs necessary for attaining that score' (p126)*

Seijts and Latham (2005) tested their ideas in a complex business simulation in which participants were asked either to attain 21% of the market share for their product (*a performance outcome goal*) or to discover three effective strategies to increase their market share (*an aspirational learning goal*). In doing so, it was discovered that individuals with the learning goals went on to increase their market share by almost twice as much as those with a performance outcome goal. More than this, the participants with the learning goals were more confident that they could master the task and demonstrated greater commitment. Although no equivalent evidence appears to exist in relation to therapeutic goals, the principles articulated by Seijts and Latham add credibility to measuring a person's progress using the Model of Human Occupation's dimensions of engagement (Kielhofner and Forsyth 2008, Pépin 2017).

Achievable

It has been found that a child's self-identified goals can be as achievable as those identified by their parents (Vroland-Nordstrand et al. 2016), and that although therapists may worry that non-achievement may affect their client's wellbeing adversely, clients themselves do not always share these concerns (Scobbie et al. 2014). So do therapists need reminding to make goals achievable? Interestingly the A in SMART is considered by some to mean Aspirational (McPherson et al. 2014), which is entirely different from being Achievable or Attainable. Furthermore, it has been noted that aspirational goals may actually help to sustain motivation (Bright et al. 2011) and that people may still achieve positive outcomes even when they fail to achieve the end goal (Levack et al. 2006b). In practise, therefore, therapists have been found to balance their own sense of what might be realistic with their clients' ideas of what might be achievable, in order to preserve their hope and dreams (Leroy et al. 2015).

If aspirational goals are set, then it undoubtedly becomes harder to know whether the person will ever achieve them, and for this reason, Kathryn McPherson et al.

(2014) conclude that rehabilitation goals need to include an element that focuses on learning development or 'the discovery of strategies and skills necessary for goal attainment' (Latham 2003). They point out that rehabilitation is rarely just about simple task completion and contend that goal setting and goal striving should be viewed as part of the therapeutic process, and not just as a means to an end. Learning is an achievement in its own right.

Box 9.7 Author's note

by Dr Rob Brooks

Along with specifying the process of change, you can specify any other conditions (or supports) that would make a goal more achievable. This may involve limiting the goal to a particular setting, or stipulating that the goal will be achieved with a certain level of support. For instance, the goal might state that the person will plan how to make friends in a particular social setting, or that a person will practise shopping in their local corner shop before they attempt shopping in a larger supermarket. However, whereas specifying a setting is not always necessary, it is essential to negotiate and stipulate the degree of support that the person will receive in order to achieve a goal. If the person expects to complete a stage of change independently, then this should be stated, but more often than not there are people who can assist the person with their progress, and negotiating the level of support can be very reassuring for the person.

Care should be taken to describe the level of support expected if the goal is to be measured. If the plan was simply to advise or encourage or prompt the person, but the therapist goes on to provide more intensive support, for example instructing the person or accompanying them or supervising them, then the goal will not be achieved as expected. There is also an ulterior motive for wording the level of support carefully if the level of support is to be provided by the occupational therapists, as the wording can be used to showcase the breadth of occupational therapy intervention from the simple provision of 'feedback' to the more demanding provision of 'coaching' (de las Heras de Pablo et al. 2017), or from gentle 'encouragement' to extensive 'collaboration' (Taylor 2008).

Relevant

If A stands for Achievable, then it makes more sense if R is Relevant as opposed to being Realistic, given that Realistic and Achievable are virtually synonymous, and the idea that goals should be relevant appears to be indisputable. Indeed, it is accepted that occupational goals should: be meaningful to the clients (Kolehmainen et al. 2012); emphasise the person's own needs, concerns, and priorities (Waller 2015); and reflect the major occupational changes sought by clients (Park 2009). This suggests that they should be in line with the person's life goals, especially since there is evidence that progress towards life goals is linked to wellbeing (Armstrong 2008). Also, it follows that when long-term goals need to be broken down into smaller goals (Annesi 2002), these should continue to capture the person's priorities and concerns, rather than being reduced to the more simple interventions prescribed during the process of therapy (Park 2009) (see Figure 9.1).

Of course, goals should also be relevant to the therapist's scope of practice, and contemporary literature calls for occupational therapists to negotiate goals that are occupation focused (Page et al. 2015). In practice, however, occupational therapists may be constrained by the expectations of the healthcare providers who employ them (Spencer et al. 1999) or be influenced by their own intervention priorities (Ribeiro et al. 2016). For instance, occupational therapists in physical healthcare settings have reported that they concentrate on the performance of activities of daily living and the skills required to perform these rather than the wider aspects of occupational participation and any associated psychosocial components (Spencer et al. 1999). Meanwhile, occupational therapists in mental health settings have been found to prioritise issues relating to their clients' habits and daily living routines when their clients would have preferred to focus on problem-solving. This last example gives strength to the arguments outlined above, which state that goals should focus on learning rather than behavioural achievement.

Timed

The one element of the SMART acronym that is rarely challenged is that it should be Timed, or Time-bound, Timely, or that it should stipulate a Timeframe or a Timeline. The most obvious reason for timing a goal is to prompt the therapist to measure whether the goal has been met at this point, as there would be no point in writing a measurable goal if it were never measured. It could also be argued that people are motivated to respond to deadlines and that by setting timeframes the therapist is able to give regular feedback to enhance motivation. On the other hand, it should be noted that deadlines could serve to reduce intrinsic motivation (Ryan and Deci 2000) and views can differ as to whether putting timeframes on goals is desirable for the individuals concerned (Brown et al. 2013), especially when people are not used to setting goals to be achieved by certain dates (Spencer et al. 1999).

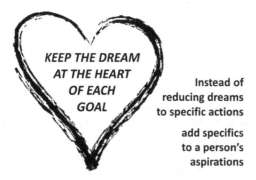

Figure 9.1 Illustration adapted from an online video: 'Constructing measurable occupational goals using the Model of Human Occupation'.
    (*Source: Parkinson and Gray 2016*).

A particular problem with setting a timeframe is that therapists sometimes only focus on short-term gains to be made during an admission or episode of care (Spencer et al. 1999). Typically, if the overarching goal of the service is to facilitate timely and safe hospital discharge, then goals are negotiated to fit this framework (Welch and Forster 2003). The risk is that goals that can be achieved in a short timeframe are focused on at the expense of longer-term goals (Levack et al. 2011). In addition, a person's achievements in the hospital might not be maintained when they leave the hospital and encounter different challenges. Either way, these problems suggest that timeframes might benefit from extending beyond the time allotted in therapy to encourage individuals to work towards their aspirational goals.

Box 9.8   Author's note

by Dr Rob Brooks

As with all the other components of a goal, the timeframe can be negotiated with the individual. Of course, it can only be negotiated after the focus of therapy has been agreed, after the expected level of change has been specified, and after the level of support has been stipulated. Once these details are in place, it becomes so much easier to foresee the timescale required. So, ask your client what they think would be a reasonable timeframe, and if an earlier timescale is preferred you can always renegotiate the level of occupational engagement or the degree of support to increase the chances of success.

Although agreeing the timeframe is the last thing to be negotiated, I would always place the timeframe in prime position when writing a goal. This helps everyone to be aware of the time limits, and will help you to remember when each goal needs to be reviewed and evaluated.

How to write a goal that TICKS all the boxes

On reflection, the SMART acronym remains a useful guide to the qualities of a measurable goal, if one interprets it as follows:

- **S** is for the inclusion of Specific *components*
- **M** is for Measuring the process of *learning*
- **A** is for making the Aspirational goals Achievable by negotiating *a level of support*
- **R** is for being Relevant to the *Key issues* identified during the formulation process
- **T** is for Timed

However, although the SMART acronym describes the *qualities* of a measurable goal, it does not specify the specific *components* that are required, with the exception of a timeframe. In other words, it does not provide clinicians with a set format for writing a measurable goal, and another acronym is needed for this.

The example goals in the third section of this book have all been written in the same format and would have been negotiated in the same order.

Table 9.1 Top tips for negotiating goals

- Agree with the formulation and the focus of therapy in relation to three or four key issues

    o If a formulation is not in place, you can still offer exploratory interventions and agree initial aims

- Negotiate one goal for each issue and renegotiate successive goals, as they are reviewed

    o If an issue comprises several activities – e.g., 'personal care activities' – then consider reducing the initial goal to focus on one activity at a time, but specify this by writing e.g., 'one personal care activity (i.e., bathing)' and not simply 'bathing', to be clear that successive goals will need to focus on the other remaining personal care activities

- Keep the person's dream at the heart of each goal

    o Reconsider what it means to have 'specific goals'
    o Add specifics to the person's hopes and aspirations instead of reducing the person's long-term dreams to specific targets (based on the person's observed actions or your interventions)
    o Specify the key occupational words in each issue, and use these in the initial goals and all successive goals
    o Whenever possible, write goals for the person to achieve – referring to their name
    o Consider writing goals in the first or second person singular ('I' or 'you')

- Negotiate the specific components of a goal with key others

    o If a person does not see the need for setting goals, then explain why you need to set them to measure your own effectiveness, and continue to provide feedback about the person's progress
- Measure the process of change by negotiating/specifying the expected level of lasting change using the Model of Human Occupation's dimensions of engagement

    o The levels may be referred to in the future tense ('the person will ...') or the future perfect tense ('the person will have ...')

- Make goals more achievable by always negotiating/specifying the degree of support and by sometimes agreeing specific settings

    o Do not write 'with the support of' someone, as this does not specify the degree of support
    o Support is likely to be given by the therapist or a member of support staff that the therapist can delegate to. If other people are to provide support, this should be negotiated beforehand
    o Consider writing the names of the people who give the support rather than their professional title

- Negotiate a specific timeframe

    o Ask the person about their preferred timescale
    o Set the timeframe to fit the time preferred and/or the time available – renegotiating the level of change or the degree of support if necessary
    o Where possible, negotiate a different timeframe for each goal, as this reduces the stress of meeting multiple deadlines

(*Continued*)

Table 9.1 (Continued)

o Specify timeframes in terms of weeks or months or dates, or even occasionally in days, but do not set deadlines according to the number of therapeutic sessions as this is not always within the person's control and rarely clear to others

o Negotiate the timeframe last, when everything else has been negotiated, but write it first in the goal to help everyone remember when the goal will be reviewed

1. an occupational formulation is agreed, from which the *Key issues* are negotiated
2. the *Individual* responsible for addressing each issue is negotiated - usually this will be the person portrayed in the formulation, but occasionally it might be a caregiver, a family member, a support worker, a team, or even the occupational therapist
3. the inner *Change expected* is negotiated regarding the process of learning – mostly using the dimensions of engagement that featured in the Model of Human Occupation (ed. Taylor 2017)
4. any *Supports* are negotiated - these always include a level of social support unless the individual is expected to achieve the goal independently, and this support is often provided by the occupational therapist. The goals may also include support in terms of the physical environment being restricted to a particular setting
5. only when all the above components have been negotiated, can a timeframe be negotiated

Although the timeframe is the last component to be negotiated, it is the first component to be written in the goal (see Table 9.1), so that everyone is clear about when the goal will be reviewed, and the whole goal is written in the following order

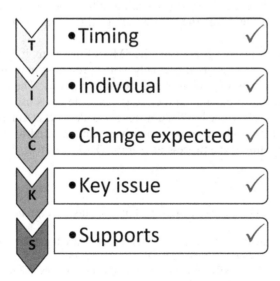

Figure 9.2 Method for writing goals using the acronym TICKS.

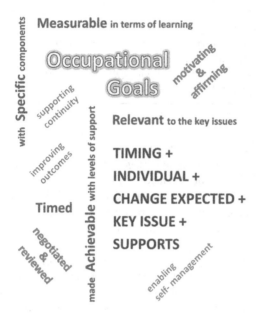

Figure 9.3 Occupational goals.

- Timeframe – the specific time by which the goal will be achieved
- Individual – the pronoun or the name(s) specifying who is to achieve the goal
- Change expected – a verb specifying the expected level of engagement
- Key issue – the occupational issue specified during the formulation process
- Supports – the level of assistance, and a specific setting if this can be graded

... giving the acronym **TICKS** which, metaphorically-speaking, allows occupational therapists to tick each component on the list as they write each goal (see Figure 9.2).

It would appear that when practitioners write goals using the SMART acronym, it does not provide sufficient guidance as to how the goals are actually written, resulting in many practitioners writing objectives by focusing on specific targets or interventions. The acronym TICKS has been designed so that occupational therapists can write goals using a consistent format, allowing long-term goals to be broken down into smaller goals (Annesi 2002) that capture the person's priorities and concerns, rather than being reduced to the more simple interventions prescribed during the process of therapy (Park 2009).

References

Annesi JJ (2002) Goal-setting protocol in adherence to exercise by Italian adults. *Perceptual and Motor Skills*, 94(2), 453–458.

Armstrong J (2008) The benefits and challenges of interdisciplinary, client-centred goal setting in rehabilitation. *New Zealand Journal of Occupational Therapy*, 55(1), 20–25.

Arnetz JE, Almin I, Bergstrom K, Franzen Y, Nilsson H (2004) Active patient involvement in the establishment of physical therapy goals: effects on treatment outcome and quality of care. *Advances in Physiotherapy*, 6(2), 50–69.

Barnett D (1999) The rehabilitation nurse as educator. In: M Smith ed. *Rehabilitation in Adult Nursing Practice*. Edinburgh: Churchill Livingstone. 53–76.

Boa S, Duncan EAS, Haraldsdottir E, Wyke S (2014) Goal setting in palliative care: a structured review. *Progress in Palliative Care, 22(6)*, 326–333.

Bovend'Eerdt TJ, Botell RE, Wade DT (2009) Writing SMART rehabilitation goals and achieving goal attainment scaling: A practical guide. *Clinical Rehabilitation 23(4)*, 352–361.

Bowman J, Mogensen L, Marsland E, Lannin N (2015) The development, content validity and inter-rater reliability of the SMART-Goal Evaluation Method: a standardised method for evaluating clinical goals. *Australian Occupational Therapy Journal, 62(6)*, 420–427.

Brewer K, Pollock N, Wright V (2014) Addressing the challenges of collaborative goal setting with children and their families. *Physical & Occupational Therapy In Pediatrics, 34(2)*, 138–152.

Bright FA, Kayes NM, McCann CM, McPherson KM (2011) Understanding hope after stroke: a systematic review of the literature using concept analysis. *Topics in Stroke Rehabilitation, 18(5)*, 490–508.

Brown, M, Levack W, McPherson KM, Dean SG, Reed K, Weatherall M, Taylor WJ (2013) Survival, momentum, and things that make me "me": patients' perceptions of goal setting after stroke, *Disability and Rehabilitation, 36(12)*, 1020–1026.

College of Occupational Therapists [COT] (2013) *Position Statement: Occupational Therapists' Use of Standardised Outcome Measures*. London: COT

College of Occupational Therapists [COT] (2016) Goals of occupational therapy intervention. In: *Occupational Therapy Terminology Supporting Occupation-centred Practice*. London: COT. https://www.rcot.co.uk/sites/default/files/1-Overview-Occupational-therapy-language-and-SNOMED-CT-Oct2016_0.pdf.

Dekker J, de Groot V, ter Steeg AM, Vloothuis J, Holla J, Collette E, Satink T, Post L, Doodeman S, Littooij E (2020) Setting meaningful goals in rehabilitation: rationale and practical tool. *Clinical Rehabilitation, 34(1)*, 3–12.

de las Heras de Pablo CG (2011) Promotion of occupational participation: integration of the Model of Human Occupation in practice. *Israeli Journal of Occupational Therapy, 20*, E67–E88.

de las Heras de Pablo C, Parkinson S, Pépin G, Kielhofner G [posthumous] (2017) Intervention process: enabling occupational change. In RR Taylor, ed. *Kielhofner's Model of Human Occupation*. Philadelphia: Wolters Kluwer. 195–216.

Doig E, Fleming J, Cornwell PL, Kuipers P (2009) Qualitative exploration of a client-centered, goal-directed approach to community-based occupational therapy for adults with traumatic brain injury. *American Journal of Occupational Therapy, 63(5)*, 559–568.

Duncan E (2016) *How bucket lists help the terminally ill – and those around them. The Conversation*, December.

Flink M, Bertilsson A-S, Johansson U, Guidetti S, Tham K, von Kock L (2016) Training in client-centeredness enhances occupational therapist documentation on goal setting and client participation in goal setting in the medical records of people with stroke. *Clinical Rehabilitation, 30(12)*, 1200–1210.

Gateley CA, Borcherding S (2012) *Documentation Manual for Occupational Therapy: Writing SOAP Notes*. 3rd ed. Thorofare, NJ: SLACK.

Garvey J, Connolly D, Boland F, Smith SM (2015) OPTIMAL, an occupational therapy led self-management support programme for people with multimorbidity in primary care: a randomized controlled trial. *BMC Family Practice 16(1)*, 59. https://www.ncbi.nlm.nih.gov/pubmed/25962515 Accessed 08/08/2019.

Herdman KA, Vandermorris S, Davidson S, Au A, Troyer AK (2018) Comparable achievement of client-identified, self-rated goals in intervention and no-intervention groups: reevaluating the use of Goal Attainment Scaling as an outcome measure. *Neuropsychological Rehabilitation, 29(10)*, 1600–1610.

Joosten AV (2015) Contemporary occupational therapy: our occupational therapy models are essential to occupation centred practice. *Australian Occupational Therapy Journal, 62(3)*, 219–222.

Kielhofner G (2009) *Conceptual Foundations of Occupational Therapy.* 4th ed. FA Davis Company, Philadelphia

Kielhofner G, Barrett L (1998) Meaning and misunderstanding in occupational forms: a study of therapeutic goal setting. *American Journal of Occupational Therapy, 52(5)*, 345–353.

Kielhofner G, Forsyth K (2008) Occupational engagement: how clients achieve change. In: G Kielhofner ed. *Model of Human Occupation: Theory and Application.* 4th ed. Baltimore: Lippincott, Williams & Wilkins, 101–109.

Kiresuk TJ, Sherman RE (1968) Goal attainment scaling: a general method for evaluating comprehensive community mental health programs. *Community Mental Health Journal, 4(6)*, 443–453.

Kolehmainen N, MacLennan G, Ternent L, Duncan EAS, Duncan EM, Ryan S, McKee L, Francis J (2012) Using shared goal setting to improve access and equity: a mixed methods study of the Good Goals intervention in children's occupational therapy. *Implementation Science.* 7:76. Accessed 08/08/2019.

Kolehmainen N, Duncan ES, Francis J (2013) Clinicians' actions associated with the successful patient care process: a content analysis of interviews with paediatric occupational therapists *Disability and Rehabilitation, 35(5)*, 388–396.

Latham GP (2003) A five-step approach to behaviour change. *Organizational Dynamics, 32(3)*, 309–318.

Law M, Pollock N, Stewart D (2004) Evidence-based occupational therapy: concepts and strategies. *New Zealand Journal of Occupational Therapy, 51(1)*, 14–22.

LeRoy K, Boyd K, De Asis K, Lee RWT, Martin R, Teachman G, Gibson BE (2015) Balancing hope and realism in family-centered care: physical therapists' dilemmas in negotiating walking goals with parents of children with Cerebral Palsy. *Physical & Occupational Therapy in Pediatrics, 35(3)*, 253–264.

Levack WMM, Taylor K, Siegert RJ, Dean SG, McPherson KM, Weatherall M (2006a) Is goal-planning in rehabilitation effective? A systematic review. *Clinical Rehabilitation, 20(9)*, 739–755.

Levack WM, Dean SG, Siegert RJ, McPherson KM (2006b) Purposes and mechanisms of goal planning in rehabilitation: the need for a critical distinction. *Disability and Rehabilitation 28(12)*, 741–749.

Levack WMM, Dean SG, Siegert RJ, McPherson KM (2011) Navigating patient-centered goal setting in inpatient stroke rehabilitation: how clinicians control the process to meet perceived professional responsibilities. *Patient Education and Counselling, 85(2)*, 206–213.

Levack WMM, Weatherall M, Hay Smith EJC, Dean SG, McPherson K, Siegert RJ (2015) Goal setting and strategies to enhance goal pursuit for adults with acquired disability participating in rehabilitation (Review). *Cochrane Database of Systematic Reviews*, (7). DOI: 10. 1002/14651858.CD009727.pub2.

Levack WM, Weatherall M, Hay-Smith JC, Dean SG, McPherson K, Siegert RJ (2016) Goal setting and strategies to enhance goal pursuit in adult rehabilitation: summary of a Cochrane systematic review and meta-analysis. *European Journal of Physical and Rehabilitation Medicine, 52(3)*, 400–416.

Levack WMM (2018) Goal setting in rehabilitation. In: S Lennon, G Ramdharry, G Verheyden, *Physical Management for Neurological Conditions* 4th ed. Poland: Elsevier. 91–109.

Linhorst DM, Hamilton G, Young E, Eckert A (2002) Opportunities and barriers to empowering people with severe mental illness through participation in treatment planning. *Social Work, 47(4)*, 425–434.

McPherson KM, Kayes NM, Kerston P (2014) MEANING as a smarter approach to Goals in Rehabilitation. In: RJ Siegert, WMM Levack eds. *Rehabilitation Goal Setting: Theory, Practice and Evidence.* Boca Raton: CRC Press. 105–122.

Page J, Roos K, Bänziger A, Margot-Cattin I, Agustoni S, Rossini E, Meichtry A, Meyer S (2015) Formulating goals in occupational therapy: state of the art in Switzerland. *Scandinavian Journal of Occupational Therapy, 22(6)*, 403–415.

Park S (2009) Goal-setting in occupational therapy: a client-centred perspective. In: Duncan EAS ed. *Skills for Practice in Occupational Therapy*. London, UK: Churchill Livingstone. 105–122.

Parkinson S (2014) *Recovery Through Activity: Increasing Participation In Everyday Life.* London: Speechmark Publishing.

Parkinson S, Gray E (2016) Constructing measurable goals using the Model of Human Occupation. [Online video]. Available at https://www.youtube.com/watch?v=HjY5_sAt2d8 Accessed 08/04/2020.

Parkinson S, Shenfield M, Reece K, Elliott J (2011) Enhancing clinical reasoning through the use of evidence-based assessments, robust case formulations and measurable goals. *British Journal of Occupational Therapy 74(3)*, 148–152.

Paterson M, Summerfield-Mann L (2006) Clinical Reasoning. In: EAS Duncan ed. *Foundations for Practice in Occupational Therapy*. Edinburgh, Scotland: Churchill Livingstone. 315–335.

Pépin G (2017) Occupational engagement: how clients achieve change. In: RR Taylor ed. *Kielhofner's Model of Human Occupation*. 5th ed. Philadelphia: Wolters Kluwer. 187–194.

Randall K, McEwan I (2000) Writing patient-centred functional goals. *Physical Therapy, 80(12)*, 1197–1203.

Ribeiro J, Rodrigues PB, Marques A, Firmino A, Lavos S (2016) Occupational therapy's intervention on mental health: perception of clients and occupational therapists about intervention priorities. In: A Costa, L Reis, F Neri de Sousa, A Moreira, D Lamas D, eds. *Computer Supported Qualitative Research. Studies in Systems, Decision and Control*, vol 71. Switzerland: Springer.

Richard LF, Knis-Matthews L (2010) Are we really client-centered? Using the Canadian Occupational Performance measure to see how the client's goals connect with the goals of the occupational therapist. *Occupational Therapy in Mental Health, 26(1)*, 51–66.

Royal College of Occupational Therapists (RCOT) (2018) *Keeping Records: Guidance for Occupational Therapists.* 4th ed. London, UK: RCOT.

Ryan RM, Deci EL (2000) Self-determination theory and the facilitation of intrinsic motivation, social development, and well-being. *American Psychologist, 55(1)*, 68–78.

Saito Y, Tomori K, Sawada T, Takahashi S, Nakatsuka S, Sugawara H, Yaginuma T, Sato T, Kumagai A, Nishimaki S, Hirano Y, Wauke Y, Weatherall M, Levack W (2019) Determining whether occupational therapy goals match between pairs of occupational therapists and their clients: a cross-sectional study. *Disability and Rehabilitation 28*, 1–6. doi: 10.1080/09638288. 2019.1643417. [Epub ahead of print]

Schell BA, Gillen G, Scaffa M, Cohn ES (2013) *Willard and Spackman's Occupational Therapy*. Philadelphia: Lippincott Williams & Wilkins.

Scobbie L, Wyke S, Dixon D, Mclean D, Duncan EAS (2013) Implementing a framework for goal setting in community based stroke rehabilitation: a process evaluation. *BMC Health Services Research*, 13:190 Accessed 08/08/2019.

Scobbie L, Duncan EA, Brady MC, Wyke S (2014) Goal setting practice in services delivering community-based stroke rehabilitation: a United Kingdom (UK) wide survey. *Disability and Rehabilitation, 37(14)*, 1291–1298.

Scott AH, Haggerty EJ (1984) Structuring goals via goal attainment scaling in occupational therapy groups in a partial hospitalisation setting. *Occupational Therapy in Mental Health, 4(2)*, 39–58.

Seijts GH, Latham GP (2005) Learning versus performance goals: when should each be used? *The Academy of Management Executive (1993–2005)*, 19(1), 124–131.

Simpson A, Coffey M, Hannigan B, Barlow S, Cohen R, Jones A, Faulkner A, Thornton A, Vseteckov J, Haddad M, Marlowe K (2017) Cross-national mixed-methods comparative case study of recovery-focusedmental health care planning and co-ordination in acute inpatient mental healthsettings (COCAPP-A). *Health Services and Delivery Research*, 5(26). 10.3310/hsdr05260.

Spencer J, Hersch G, Eschenfelder V, Fournet J, Murray-Gerzik M (1999) Outcomes of protocol-based and adaptation-based occupational therapy interventions for low-income elderly persons on a transitional unit. *American Journal of Occupational Therapy*, 53(2), 159–170.

Tang Yan HS, Clemson LM, Jarvis F, Laver K (2014) Goal setting with caregivers of adults in the community: a mixed methods systematic review. *Disability and Rehabilitation*, 36(23), 1943–1963.

Taylor RR (2008) *The Intentional Relationship: Occupational Therapy and Therapeutic Use of Self*. Philadelphia: FA Davis.

Taylor RR, ed. (2017) *Kielhofner as Model of Human Occupation. 5th ed.* Philadelphia: Wolters Kluwer.

Turner-Stokes, L (2009) Goal Attainment Scaling (GAS) in rehabilitation: A practical guide. *Clinical Rehabilitation*, 23, 362–370. doi:10.1177/0269215508101742.

Vroland-Nordstrand K, Eliasson AC, Jacobsson H, Johansson U, Krumlinde-Sundholm L (2016) Can children identify and achieve goals for intervention? A randomized trial comparing two goal-setting approaches. *Developmental Medicine and Child Neurology*, 58(6), 589–596.

Waller P (2015) *Occupational Therapy Goals during acute discharge for older adults*. Sydney: Unpublished thesis https://ses.library.usyd.edu.au/bitstream/2123/14208/1/Waller_Paige_Thesis_Submission_e-scholarship.pdf Accessed 08/08/2019.

Welch A, Forster SA (2003) Clinical audit of the outcome of occupational therapy assessment and negotiated patient goals in the acute setting. *British Journal of Occupational Therapy*, 66(8), 363–368.

Weidenbohm K, Parsons M, Dixon R (2005) Goal attainment scaling: a tool for use in evaluation of services for older people. *New Zealand Journal of Occupational Therapy*, 52(2), 9–14.

Wong SR, Fisher G (2015) Comparing and using occupation-focused models. *Occupational Therapy In Health Care*, 29(3), 297–315.

World Federation of Occupational Therapists, von Zweck C, Alchouron C, Brandis S, Bressler S, Buchanan H, Clouston T, Cox C, Moreno L, Reistetter T, Zur A (2019) *Development of a Quality Indicator Framework for occupational therapy. World Federation of Occupational Therapists Bulletin*, 75:1, 3–10.

Part III

Example occupational formulations and goals

I Occupational Therapy in a paediatric service

– an example occupational formulation with measurable goals

Overview

Featuring a child who is 4 years old, the following formulation focuses on the youngest person in this book and reminds us that occupational formulations have no age limits, as we are all occupational beings. In this case, Emma is adapting to school life and this is the primary focus of the formulation. Even so, the formulation manages to give a rounded picture of her identity outside of school, by starting with her home life and her relationship with her baby brother.

Also, although the formulation has been written primarily for the benefit of the teaching staff and Emma's parents, the therapist still avoids a great deal of technical language. Not only are Emma's own words quoted in the identity section, but simpler language is used to express the key issues and compose the Summary statement. The result is a formulation for the whole team, including goals and actions that involve Emma, the occupational therapist, the teaching staff, and Emma's parents.

Notice how:

- Emma's strengths and limitations are not listed, but are instead woven into a narrative
- themes introduced in the identity section are followed through into the competence section. For example:

  - o loves baby brother → is a fantastic little helper
  - o happy and confident at home → now quieter when getting ready for school
  - o 'Wobbly' and feels tired → mostly gets around indoors by supporting herself on furniture, and uses a walker for longer distances
  - o has made a good friend → play date is being planned
  - o enjoys 'anything with numbers' → is good with numbers
  - o proud of writing skills → uses pencil grip
  - o feels sad when does not get things right → becomes tearful and needs reassurance

- the summary refers to

  - o *not getting things right*, rather than 'feeling frustrated'
  - o *taking part*, rather than 'participating';
  - o *feeling less tired* rather than 'conserving energy'
  - o *calming down when upset* – a phrase from the Child Occupational Self Assessment (Kramer et al. 2014) – rather than more technical phrases such as 'self-soothing'

DOI: 10.4324/9781003046301-10

Introduction

Emma is a 4½-year-old girl who has cerebral palsy which mainly affects her legs. She has no significant learning disabilities. An occupational therapist has worked with Emma and her family for several years, alongside speech and language therapists and physiotherapists. Occupational therapy is currently focused on helping Emma to adapt to school life.

Occupational assessments completed:
- Child Occupational Self Assessment (Kramer et al. 2014)
- Short Child Occupational Profile (SCOPE) (Bowyer et al. 2008)
- classroom observations and discussions with parents and teaching staff

Occupational identity

Emma loves her baby brother, Jack, and has always been happy and confident at home. She enjoys the company of her grandparents, who often looks after her when her parents were working, and is known in the therapy team for having a great imagination and an infectious sense of humour.

Emma feels shy when at school because of being 'wobbly' and because she 'did not know people' when starting school. She has already made a good friend with another girl, Isla, and they like looking at books together and playing imaginary games. She likes her teacher very much and prefers to sit near her in the classroom. She does not like going outside at break time and looks forward to rainy days when she can stay inside and play quietly.

Emma enjoys most of the lessons, especially 'anything with numbers', and is proud of her ability to use pens and pencils. She feels sad when she does not get things right and sometimes wants 'everyone to go away' so that she can be on her own. She does not like lessons that involve physical activity as she is not as fast as others and she feels 'so tired' when trying to keep up with her classmates. She would love to have a powered wheelchair so that she can 'whizz around'.

Occupational competence

Emma's mum says that Emma is a fantastic little helper with baby Jack and that the family has always encouraged Emma to be independent. She got on well with other children at the nursery she attended 3 days a week which was near her mum's workplace.

Although her speech is not always clear, she is able to make her needs known, and it was generally thought that Emma would cope well at school. She had already started to learn to read, was able to go to the toilet on her own, and could manage a knife and fork as well as most 4-year-olds can. She mostly gets around indoors by supporting herself on furniture, and uses a walker for longer distances.

It has been noticed that Emma is sometimes quieter than usual when getting ready to go to school, but soon becomes livelier when she sees her friend, Isla, at the school gates. Her parents have chatted with Isla's mum and hope to invite Isla over for a play date soon. Once at school, Emma is normally cheerful but can be tearful at times – usually when she is frustrated or tired. She then needs plenty of reassurance from the classroom teaching assistant before she can refocus on activities.

Emma is good at numbers, uses a pencil grip to help her write, and perhaps would be less tired if there was greater postural support to help her work at a desk. The classroom itself is cramped but the school has good level access throughout and a toilet that Emma can access with her walker. The playground is large and Emma's teacher is keen to think of ways to support Emma to cope in this space and to take part in physical activities. She understands that Emma should be encouraged to be as active as possible, and that Emma's manual wheelchair could be brought from home if she were to go on school trips.

Key occupational issues

- taking part in organised physical activities
- working at a desk
- making the most of break times
- calming down when upset

Summary statement

Emma is a friendly girl who loves her baby brother, likes books and imaginary play, and enjoys lots of school lessons, especially 'anything with numbers'.

Emma uses a walker at school and gets tired when trying to keep up with her classmates and upset when she cannot do things right. Thought needs to be given to how she can best take part in organised physical activities and feel less tired when working at her desk, and encouragement is required to help her make the most of break times (with best friend Isla) and calm herself down when upset.

Initial goals and interventions

1a. Over the next 2 weeks, Emma and the occupational therapist will plan how she can best take part in organised physical activities, in discussion with Emma's teacher and teaching assistant.

- occupational therapist and teacher to discuss how routine physical activities might be adapted to be more inclusive, and investigate new activities that pupils can participate in whatever their ability, with the occupational therapist providing a fact sheet
- staff to encourage Emma to be as mobile as possible, using her walker as necessary
- occupational therapist to liaise with parents to identify the best ways to inform Emma's classmates of her needs
- occupational therapist to talk with Emma and her parents to discover favourite activities

2a. Over the next 6 weeks, the occupational therapist will offer suggestions and provide equipment to help Emma explore options for working at her desk

- occupational therapist to acquire an angled surface for Emma to trial
- occupational therapist to re-assess Emma's seating needs with a view to reducing her fatigue by increasing postural support
- occupational therapist to consider chairs with armrests, posture cushions, and footrests

3a. Over the next 8 weeks, the team will identify a range of strategies to help Emma calm down when upset (and avoid upset), with advice from the occupational therapist and insights from the teaching assistant.

- teaching assistant to praise Emma when she manages well
- staff to keep a diary to determine the triggers that lead to Emma being upset, and note strategies that help her to cope
- teacher to support the whole class to think about how everyone is different and everyone has things they do well and things they find hard, and all staff to be alert to any bullying
- Emma to be allowed time to move between activities before her classmates move
- occupational therapist to observe Emma in the classroom to further assess her needs
- occupational therapist and teacher to consider whether any changes can be made to the classroom layout to increase accessibility

4a. Over the next 4 weeks, Emma's teacher will plan ways to help Emma make the most of break times with advice from the occupational therapist.

- teacher to ensure that Emma is introduced to break time supervisors and to reinforce the importance of them supporting Emma to be active
- staff to focus on helping Emma to get to know other children – during break times and in the classroom
- occupational therapist to investigate pouches to attach to a walker, allowing Emma to carry objects outside
- occupational therapist to share ideas for inclusive playgrounds

---

Box I.i   An educator's perspective

Learning this approach to occupational formulation was like finding the missing link between assessment and treatment planning, and I wish I'd learned it earlier in my career! My team had long used the Model of Human Occupation and its related assessments, but observation and audits revealed varying approaches between practising therapists. On reflection, the lack of occupational formulation and goal setting could lead to discontinuity of treatment and confusion for therapists, the team, and clients. I believe that introducing this approach to occupational formulation has the potential to strengthen the practice of the occupational therapy team, and ultimately to improve clients' occupational outcomes.

Table I.i Components of Emma's occupational identity

Roles/relationships	Big sister to baby Jack; daughter; granddaughter; known by therapy team for great imagination and infectious sense of humour; friend to Isla; classmate; pupil
Turning points (inc., changes to physical & social environments)	Born with cerebral palsy; birth of brother; moving from nursery near mother's workplace to start school
Interests	Likes looking at books and imaginary play with friend; enjoys lots of lessons, especially 'anything with numbers'
Volition *(inc., appraisal of ability, expectation of success, values, choices, satisfaction & goals)*	Loves baby brother; enjoys the company of grandparents; happy and confident at home; feels shy because of being 'wobbly' and not knowing people; likes her teacher; looks forward to rainy days as does not like going outside at break time; feels sad when unable to get things right and sometimes wants 'everyone to go away' and to be on own; does not like lessons involving physical activity; feels tired when trying to keep up with classmates; would like a powered wheelchair to whizz around in

Table I.ii Components of Emma's occupational competence

Routines	Meets friend Isla at the school gate and is having a play date soon, previously went to nursery 3 days a week
Skills	Previously got on well with other children; speech is not always clear, but is able to make needs known; can need help to refocus on tasks; mostly gets around indoors by supporting self on furniture, and uses a walker for longer distances
Performance	Fantastic little helper with baby Jack; was learning to read before starting school, able to go to the toilet on own and manage a knife and fork; sometimes quieter than usual when getting ready to go to school and more lively when sees her friend; tearful when frustrated or tired; good at maths; uses pencil grip to write and may benefit from greater postural support when working at a desk
Environmental contexts	Grandparents are involved in childcare; family have always encouraged independence; mum and dad notice her mood; mum and Isla's mum are planning playdate; teaching assistant provides reassurance; the classroom is cramped; school has good level access throughout and accessible toilet; the playground is large; teacher is keen to find ways to support going outside and taking part in physical activity; manual wheelchair could be brought from home for school trips

References

Bowyer PL, Kramer J, Ploszaj A, Ross M, Schwartz O, Kielhofner G, Kramer K (2008) *The Short Child Occupational Profile (SCOPE) Version 2.2*. Chicago: University of Illinois.

Kramer J, ten Velden M, Kafkes A, Basu, S, Federico J, Kielhofner G (2014) *Child Occupational Self Assessment (OSA) Version 2.2*. Chicago: University of Illinois.

II Occupational Therapy in a children's mental health service

– an example occupational formulation with measurable goals

Overview

Although most formulations are completed after a period of assessment and before the intervention starts in earnest, occupational therapists may well initiate activities as part of the assessment process, before clear goals have been set. In this case, the occupational therapist has already invited Lucy to take part in art-based activities. This is because occupational therapists learn a great deal about a person using occupation-based assessment methods – exploring how a person responds to invitations to participate in activities. When activities are used for assessment purposes, one might call them 'exploratory interventions' where the boundary between assessment and intervention is blurred. These exploratory interventions may or may not continue after a formulation has been reached, and the formulation stage offers an opportunity to rethink everything that has occurred and decide on a way forward.

It is also worth noting that although most goals will indicate a level of support that will be provided, it is perfectly possible for individuals to complete some goals without any further help, especially during the later stages of therapy. In this example, once the goals have been negotiated, Lucy's parents are deemed sufficiently able to accomplish one of the goals on their own. Rather than simply omitting any reference to the level of support, which might be interpreted as an act of forgetfulness, the goal clearly states that it is to be completed independently.

Notice how:
- the views of Lucy's parents are represented in the identity section – their sense that Lucy has always been 'quirky', and their hope for the future
- the routines of the family are included in the competence section – with the parents getting up early in the morning, and the family eating at irregular times
- exploratory intervention, in the form of art-based sessions, has started before the goals have been negotiated
- the findings of the Paediatric Volitional Questionnaire (Basu et al. 2008) provide the occupational therapist with detailed descriptions of Lucy's positive volitional behaviours – showing curiosity and showing a willingness to try new things
- the key occupational issues are for Lucy *and* her family
- the fourth goal is for Lucy's parents to complete independently, without any external support
- many of the actions/interventions associated with each goal are to be completed by the occupational therapist or Lucy's parents, rather than Lucy herself

---

DOI: 10.4324/9781003046301-11

Introduction

Lucy is a 12-year-old girl who has recently been diagnosed with autism. She was referred to the Child and Adolescent Mental Health team because of acute problems, at a time when she was not sleeping, and her family was at 'crisis point'. She was allocated to the occupational therapist to support issues relating to school attendance and family life.

Occupational assessments completed:
- Paediatric Volitional Questionnaire (Basu et al. 2008)
- informal interviews with Lucy and her parents

Occupational identity

Lucy lives with her parents (Amanda and Dave) and a younger sister, Hannah. She had a typical birth and early childhood, met all of her developmental milestones, and seemed to enjoy everyday family life – holidays, days out, family time, games, hobbies (photography and arts crafts), and attending various clubs.

On reflection, Lucy's parents recognise that she has always been 'a little quirky' and rigid in her thoughts and activities. Until Lucy's diagnosis of autism, Lucy's parents had no explanation for her difficulties, but recognised that they started when she moved from a small rural primary school to a large suburban high school. It seems that she became overwhelmed and her preferences became ever more limited; she started to express reluctance to attend school, she only liked certain foods, and she did not want to sleep in her bedroom. Lucy also started to express anger towards her parents and her sister, and stopped caring about her appearance.

The diagnosis of autism was unexpected by Lucy's parents and for some time they were unable to envisage a time when Lucy would be able to do anything for herself. They now hope that she will be able to return to education at some point in the future and remain keen to support Lucy in any way that they can, while wanting to maintain a sense of 'normal family life' for Hannah. Meanwhile, Lucy still finds any talk about school distressing, but she does not want to be 'like this' and would like to go outside and take photographs one day.

Occupational competence

Lucy had friends when she was at primary school and appeared to flourish. When she started to withdraw from school and her usual activities, her parents worked hard to accommodate her concerns and began to adapt their family life. At one point they were getting up at 5 am to encourage and persuade Lucy to go to school, before Amanda gave up her work as an administrator 6 months ago to homeschool Lucy. The family now tends to eat at irregular times, and there have been occasions when they have driven out in the middle of the night to buy specific foods for Lucy.

Over the last 4 months, Lucy began refusing to go to bed, and she stopped washing her body or hair, and brushing her teeth. Her behaviours became violent towards her parents and sister, and attempts to school Lucy at home stopped. At the point of referral, she was spending all her time on the living room sofa under a duvet, shouting at her parents to go away when they asked her how she was feeling.

Lucy's sleep is still erratic and she has difficulty engaging in conversation about her future needs and calming herself down when upset. Her hair is still matted but she gets dressed occasionally and is currently managing to engage in art-based activities for half-an-hour at a time. During these sessions, she is task-directed and demonstrates an ability to practise new skills. She still finds it difficult to use imagination and respond to challenges, but shows curiosity and is willing to try new things.

Key occupational issues for Lucy and her family

- doing things she likes
- looking after herself
- having a family life
- continuing with her education

Summary statement

Lucy enjoyed friendships and family life when she was at primary school – holidays, days out, family games, and hobbies.

She is learning to do things that she likes again, including photography, and arts and crafts. Looking after herself is still a struggle, but she is sleeping better, and she now gets dressed occasionally. Her family is committed to supporting her and re-gaining a family life in which Lucy is able to manage her emotions, participate in family meals, and sleep in her own room. Eventually, it will be important for Lucy to continue her education perhaps at a smaller school.

Initial goals and interventions

1a. Over the next 6 weeks, Lucy will practise activities that she likes, facilitated by the occupational therapist

- occupational therapist to bring art resources to Lucy in her home and plan graded activities
- occupational therapist to provide positive feedback and assist Lucy to recognise her feelings, especially when she feels calm and happy
- occupational therapist and Lucy to plan a photography project
- occupational therapist to work with Lucy to complete an Interest Checklist

2a. Over the next 4 weeks, Lucy will negotiate the help that she needs to look after herself with encouragement and suggestions from the occupational therapist

- occupational therapist to identify sensory issues affecting Lucy's participation in activities of daily living
- occupational therapist to identify an accessible hairdressing service

- occupational therapist to provide education to Lucy's parents regarding sleep hygiene and liaise with psychiatrist regarding possible medical interventions to improve sleep
- occupational therapist to provide reassurance and offer opportunities for Lucy to describe how she wants to be, possibly using the Child Occupational Self-Assessment
- occupational therapist to advise on ways to manage stresses when engaging in self-care activities and suggest self-care activities that Lucy might enjoy

3a. Over the next 8 weeks, Lucy's parents will identify ways to help Lucy participate in family life, with advice from the occupational therapist

- Lucy's parents to plan everyday activities with advice from the occupational therapist on how to introduce changes and manage transitions
- Lucy's parents to keep a diary noting Lucy's responses
- Lucy's parents to plan quality time with Hannah and seek support from friends and family members

4a. Over the next 3 months, Lucy's parents will independently explore options for Lucy continuing her education

- Lucy's parents to arrange to meet with her teachers to review their observations and any recommendations
- Lucy's parents to investigate alternative schools in the local area
- occupational therapist to initiate discussion of Lucy's fears with her, and identify her strengths and limitations in pursuing her education

---

Box II.i A manager's perspective

Within the mental health service that I manage, all the occupational therapists have been trained to develop occupational formulations and action plans, as agreed when goal planning with the service user. The formulations are presented to the multi-disciplinary team in case conferences in both hospital and community mental health teams, where their focus on identity, valued occupations, and goals reinforces recovery-based practice of hope and choice.

The formulations are also referred to in professional occupational therapy supervision; and by reviewing them when the occupational process seems confused, feels frustrating, or is not progressing, I have found that clear goals can be agreed for all.

Finally, should an occupational therapist move to another service, the occupational formulation and goals provide a summary of work to date, ensuring that no goals are lost in the transfer of care. They also afford a very positive place to start with a person – ensuring that the first meeting focuses on the actions and supports needed to meet the person's ongoing goals.

Table II.i Components of Lucy's occupational identity

Roles/relationships	Daughter, sister, pupil, club member; parents were unable to envisage progress – now hoping she may return to school and wanting to maintain a normal family life
Turning points (inc., changes to physical & social environments)	Moving from small rural primary school to a large suburban high school
Interests	Holidays, family time, games, photography, arts & crafts
Volition *(inc., appraisal of ability, expectation of success, values, choices, satisfaction & goals)*	Quirky, rigid, overwhelmed; preferences became limited – liked certain foods only; reluctant to attend school; did not want to sleep in her bedroom; started to express anger towards parents and sister; stopped caring about appearance; finds talk of school distressing; does not want to be like this; would like to go outside and take photographs one day

Table II.ii Components of Lucy's occupational competence

Routines	Withdrew from school; eating at irregular times; stopped washing and brushing teeth or hair; spending all her time under a duvet; erratic sleep
Skills	Difficulty engaging in conversation and calming self down; task-directed during therapy sessions; demonstrates ability to learn
Performance	Had friends; was flourishing; refusing to go to bed; shouting at parents; violent; gets dressed occasionally; managing art-based activities in half-an-hour therapy sessions; difficulty using imagination and responding to challenges but shows curiosity and is willing to try new things
Environmental contexts	Family life has been adapted – parents getting up at 5 am and driving out in the middle of the night; home-schooling has stopped

Reference

Basu S, Kafkes A, Schatz R, Kiraly A, Kielhofner G (2008) *The Pediatric Volitional Questionnaire (PVQ) Version 2.1*. Chicago: University of Illinois.

III Occupational Therapy in an adolescent mental health service

– an example occupational formulation with measurable goals

Overview

Whereas the client in the previous formulation was referred to the occupational therapist because of behavioural issues that were clearly affecting occupational participation, Mick was referred because of anxiety and depression stemming from childhood neglect and abuse. It would have been easy for an occupational therapist to focus on helping him to manage his symptoms and to focus exclusively on psychological therapy techniques. The occupational formulation provides an opportunity to make a case for focusing on things that are practical, everyday, and even ordinary – the things that really matter if Mick's life is to move forward. This does not mean that the occupational therapist does not help Mick to manage his anxiety or use psychological strategies to help him manage his negative thoughts. He can do all this and more, but he makes a deliberate choice to measure the success of these interventions by the occupational changes that they produce. In doing so, he builds evidence for occupational therapy's unique contribution.

The second person singular – 'you' – is used throughout the formulation to great effect. The whole formulation reads more like a letter than a clinical document; a letter in which the occupational therapist is checking out his understanding and helping Mick to make sense of his life. And although Mick is still only 16, it is clear that his life has already taken many twists and turns which impact his sense of occupational identity and provide the backdrop to his occupational competence. Both sections are written in a flowing narrative style which prepares the way for agreeing the more formal goals and interventions that follow.

Notice how:

- after the introduction, Mick is always referred to as 'you'
- the formulation includes beautiful details that bring the narrative to life – from the type of comic book films that Mick loves, to the name and breed of his foster parents' dog
- the findings of the Assessment of Communication and Interaction Skills provide the occupational therapist with evidence of positive social behaviour – collaborating with others to complete tasks
- the name of the occupational therapist is referred to in the interventions, emphasising a human connection
- so many different turning points feature in the components of Mick's occupational identity

---

DOI: 10.4324/9781003046301-13

Introduction

Mick is 16 years old. He was referred to the Child and Adolescent Mental Health Service by the sexual exploitation team and allocated to the occupational therapist for help in managing his anxiety and depression.

Occupational assessments completed:
- Occupational Circumstances Assessment Interview and Rating Scale (OCAIRS) (Forsyth et al. 2005)
- Assessment of Communication and Interaction Skills (ACIS) (Forsyth et al. 1998)

Occupational identity

You think of yourself as a caring person, who loves dogs, and who would like to use your experiences to help others. Eventually, you would like to earn enough money to buy a house of your own and look after your mum.

You were brought up by your mum and her partner, whom you believed to be your biological dad. Both had drug and alcohol problems, and you describe your early years as being, 'loving but a bit of a mess'. Your family were 'on the breadline' and you remember not always having enough to eat, few family outings, and no holidays. You spent a lot of your childhood watching TV – developing a love for comic book films, including the X-Men and the Avengers – and you would love to be a film director or a comic book artist. Although you did attend school, you were often jealous of your classmates, and would fight and then fall out with any friends that you had made.

At the age of 12, your mum and her partner went into rehab and at this time you found out that your mother's partner was your 'real' dad's brother. Although this was a shock, you started to dream about having a more stable life with a new family. You were reunited with your biological father, who lived with his female partner and their two children, and decided to move in with them. It was during this stay that you were groomed and sexually abused by a neighbour who has since been convicted. You do not want to talk about this period of your life and now find it difficult to trust others.

You have little confidence in your abilities but are motivated to turn your life around. You have started to attend college to study Health and Social Care, and would like to pursue a career in this field.

Occupational competence

You are currently living with foster parents (Teresa and Steve) who own a greyhound called Jet. You have consistently respected their advice and they say that you often help out around the house. You also take Jet for walks and spend time with him when you feel 'mixed up'. Meanwhile, your birth mother has continued to struggle with her addictions. You phone her once a week and have visited her twice in the last 6 months.

You experience negative thoughts of self-blame and still have times when you 'snap' at others – sometimes when they make requests, and sometimes when you doubt their friendliness. These verbal outbursts are short-lived and are usually followed by you withdrawing to your room to watch fantasy films and read comic books.

Your attendance at college is irregular and you benefit from encouragement to complete your course work. You have experienced panic attacks when using buses to travel to college and will then get off the bus and walk around the town for hours at a time. Despite missing classes, the coursework that you have produced has been satisfactory and you are beginning to develop an effective study routine. You still have difficulty initiating and sustaining social conversation, but have shown that you can work with others to complete tasks.

Key occupational issues

*   coping with bus journeys
*   maintaining social conversation
*   completing your college course
*   finding a social outlet for your interests

Summary statement

You love comic books and films, find comfort in being with your foster parents' dog, Jet, and are studying Health and Social Care at college.

You are sometimes overcome by panic attacks when traveling to college and have difficulty trusting others, so you would like to be able to cope with bus journeys and to initiate and sustain social conversations. Although you sometimes miss classes, your study skills are improving, and completing your chosen college course is important to you. Finding a social outlet would be beneficial too – one in which you can be with others who share the same interests.

Initial goals and interventions

1a. Over the next 6 weeks, you will practise a range of strategies to help you cope with bus journeys, with advice and instruction from Paul, your occupational therapist

   *   Paul to teach anxiety management strategies, including breathing techniques, distraction techniques, postural relaxation, and ways to challenge negative thoughts
   *   Paul to accompany Mick on a bus journey from his home to college, and analyse triggers for panic attacks
   *   Mick to practise techniques at home and on the bus

2a. Over the next 2 weeks, you will identify your strengths in maintaining social conversations, with prompts and feedback from Paul

   *   Paul and Mick to share and summarise positive aspects of Mick's interaction at the end of each session
   *   Mick to ask Teresa and Steve to help him reflect on his conversational skills

3a. Over the next 8 weeks, you will plan and negotiate the support you need to complete your college course, with assistance from Paul, and your foster parents Teresa and Steve

   *   Paul to investigate support options at college
   *   Mick and Paul to discuss what helps and what does not help college attendance
   *   Mick, Teresa and Steve to arrange a meeting at college to discuss support options

4a. Over the next 4 weeks, you will explore options for a social outlet based on your interests, with encouragement and ideas from Paul

- Paul and Mick to play a fantasy card game
- Paul to check out local opportunities for fantasy gaming
- Mick to find out about Pokémon Go

Box III.i A therapists' perspective

The process of using occupational formulation and measurable goal setting has transformed my practice. Synthesising assessment information, pulling out key areas for change, and setting goals, ensuring these goals are occupation focussed, measurable, and retain a focus on areas of change (and not the interventions), has always tested me professionally. The procedure outlined in this book provided a solution. It offers a structure to guide professional reasoning through this challenging part of the Occupational Therapy process. Used service-wide, it ensures a consistent structure which has had a positive impact on professional identity.

Although standardised occupation-focused outcome measures provide a structure and common language for the assessment phase, and there are many manualised, evidence-based interventions that provide a structure for the treatment phase, the planning phase that comes between assessment and intervention is often overlooked. Occupational formulations and measurable goals using MOHO provide the necessary structure and common language for this vital stage. In my personal experience, this process is effective, well overdue, and has been pivotal in strengthening occupation focused and person-centred practice.

Table III.i Components of Mick's occupational identity

Roles/relationships	Son/step-son, half-brother; previously classmate; now college student
Turning points (inc., changes to physical & social environments)	Early years being 'loving but a bit of a mess' due to mum and dad having addictions – not always having enough to eat, few family outings and no holidays; learning that 'dad' was an uncle; reunion with 'real' dad, and moving to live with him; being groomed and sexually abused by a neighbour who has since been convicted
Interests	Loves dogs, comic book films – X-men and Avengers
Volition *(inc., appraisal of ability, expectation of success, values, choices, satisfaction & goals)*	Caring – would like to help others in a caring career and earn enough money to look after mum; would love to be a film director; was jealous of classmates and dreamed of living with a new family; decided to live with 'real' dad; does not want to talk about abuse; finding it difficult to trust others and has little confidence

Table III.ii Components of Mick's occupational competence

Routines	Spends time with greyhound; phones mother once a week and has visited twice in the last 6 months; attendance at college is irregular
Skills	Respects advice of foster parents; still snaps at others at times though verbal outbursts are short-lived; has difficulty initiating and sustaining social conversation but can collaborate with others
Performance	Helps out around the house and takes dog for walks; withdraws to room when upset and watches films; has experienced panic attacks on buses; produces satisfactory coursework and is beginning to develop effective study routine
Environmental context	Lives with foster parents and their dog; mother continues to struggle with addictions

References

Forsyth K, Salamy M, Simon S, Kielhofner G (1998) *The Assessment of Communication and Interaction Skills (ACIS) Version 4.0.* Chicago: University of Illinois.

Forsyth K, Deshpande S, Kielhofner G, Henrikson C, Haglund L, Olson L, Skinner S, Kulkarni S (2005) *The Occupational Circumstances Assessment Interview and Rating Scale (OCAIRS) Version 4.0.* Chicago: University of Illinois.

IV Occupational Therapy in a perinatal mental health service

– an example occupational formulation with measurable goals

Overview

Formulations need to refer to the person's strengths as well as the challenges that they face, and you might imagine that it is easier to do this when a person has a history of achievement, as Jessica has in this formulation. Yet, even when a person's strengths are apparent, one needs to strike a careful balance. Emphasising a person's past strengths may serve to highlight their present difficulties unless you also record some positives about their current situation. There again, if you paint a picture that is too rosy, then someone like Jessica might feel that their worries are not being heard. And if you focus too much on the person's negative feelings and the difficulties that they are facing, you might be in danger of reinforcing them. So it is important to avoid catastrophizing their situation by using words such as 'very' or 'really' or 'extremely'. Even if Jessica felt that she had 'absolutely' no ability as a mother, and said that she was a 'total' failure, it is enough to say that she feels she has no ability and says she is a failure. You could also use the person's own words, placed in quotation marks, to make it clear when negative thoughts have been voiced by the person but in no way represent your professional opinion.

For those of you who are interested in language and the power that words have, another way in which you can emphasise positives is by starting with them, going on to describe the challenges, and then ending with positives again. This is sometimes known as a 'praise sandwich' – a way of making unpalatable truths easier to swallow. Another trick is never to start a sentence with a positive and then use the word 'but …', as this seems to negate the earlier positive. It is better simply to start a new sentence, *or* to invert the information so that the sentence starts with the negative but is followed on by a positive, which can be linked using phrases such as 'despite this …', or 'however …'.

Introduction

Jessica is a 33-year-old woman who has been admitted informally to a mother and baby unit after her health visitor raised concerns regarding Jessica's anxiety and depression, involving suicidal ideation, and feelings of estrangement from her newborn son. Once admitted, she was automatically referred to the occupational therapy service.

DOI: 10.4324/9781003046301-14

> **Notice how:**
> - Jessica has always had lots of interests, and the occupational therapist could have written something to this effect without providing any detail, but the detail is important, and so key interests are all listed'
> - 'Jessica's own words are quoted to good effect: 'this is not how it should be' – 'everyone else can look after my son better than I can'
> - 'both the identity and competence sections start and end with positives'
> - the first sentence of the last paragraph in the competence section describes a presenting difficulty, and the following sentence highlights a corresponding positive by starting with the phrase 'Despite this, …'
> - unlike many of the example formulations, this one shows how successive goals build on the initial goals
> - when analysing the components of Jessica's Occupational Identity, her volition is given prominence, and when analysing the components of her Occupational Competence, it becomes clear that her routines are as important as her performance

Occupational assessments completed:
- Occupational Self Assessment (OSA) (Baron et al. 2006)
- Occupational Circumstances Assessment and Interview Rating Scale (OCAIRS) (Forsyth et al. 2005)
- Model of Human Occupation Screening Tool (MOHOST) – Single observations (Parkinson et al. 2006)

Occupational identity

Jessica works full-time as a high school teacher, is the head of the history department, and has always held ambitions to become a Head Teacher. She is married to Sam who works shifts as a sergeant in the police force, and she describes having a 'happy and stable relationship'. Prior to the birth of Luke 5 weeks ago, the two had a number of shared hobbies including running and fell walking. Jessica also likes to dance, has a particular interest in Samba dancing, and normally enjoys pampering sessions. Jessica's friends are a mix of single professional people and parents with young children, including her older sister, who appears to her to have very successful lives and are confident parents.

Jessica has always held high standards for herself and others. She and Sam have recently renovated an old Victorian property and she takes great pride in keeping it looking immaculate. They have been together for 6 years and were hoping to have children for the past four. Luke was conceived after a second course of IVF and was a 'much-wanted baby'. Jessica is currently on maternity leave and is hoping to return to work when Luke is around 12 months old, when the new school year begins.

After a healthy pregnancy, Luke's birth was long and traumatic, resulting in an emergency caesarean section, and Jessica feeling out of control and scared that her baby would die. Having been very excited about the birth of her baby, Jessica currently feels she has no ability to be a mother and worries that Luke will not feed well or thrive if he remains in her care. Jessica says she is a failure as a mother, wife, and woman and finds great difficulty to see a positive future for herself – 'this is not how it should be' – 'everyone else can look after my son better than I can'. She is nevertheless clear that she loves Luke and wants to be able to breastfeed him and establish the bond that other mothers seem to have.

Occupational competence

Jessica is an articulate woman, educated to Master's degree level, and is usually very clear about her opinions. She worked and engaged in all her hobbies until close to Luke's birth, attending a Samba group twice weekly, and running every morning before work. She also visited a beauty salon regularly and spent many months with Sam creating a beautiful nursery in anticipation of Luke's arrival. Over the last 5 weeks, she has stopped tending to her own self-care and has declined visits from her friends who remain keen to see her and continue to send their best wishes. Jessica is not eating and drinking adequately, and is spending most of the day in her night-clothes, commenting that she has nothing to get dressed for.

Jessica's own mother is very supportive and tries to assist her daughter by taking care of the baby overnight 'so she can rest'. Sam also appears to have adapted to fatherhood well and enjoys tending to his son. He likes to spend his hours out of work looking after Luke by taking him for long walks in the pram or visiting his own parents who live nearby. Jessica has so far declined to be involved in these activities, and although polite she rarely initiates conversation or expresses any enthusiasm.

Luke appears to need to feed for long periods resulting in sore nipples for Jessica, and she becomes tearful when he cries (which is often). Despite this, and although Luke does not always sleep well, and is being investigated for reflux and milk intolerance, he is gaining weight as he should. Meanwhile, Jessica is not sleeping well and tires quickly when caring for Luke. She also experiences pain when bending and noticeably struggles to lift Luke, which may be because her scar has become infected. The risk of infection continuing is high due to reduced self-care, and cleaning of the wound is currently being monitored by health staff. Other than that, it is evident that Jessica is constantly aware of Luke's presence when he is nearby and this is currently affecting her concentration, but when on her own she remains a capable woman who is able to focus and complete tasks with encouragement.

Key occupational issues

- establishing self as a confident mother
- re-establishing self-care
- regaining physical fitness
- rediscovering motivation for interests

Summary statement

Jessica gave birth to her 'much wanted' baby Luke 5 weeks ago. She is the head of a history department at her school, happily married to Sam, and usually enjoys fell-running, samba dancing, and home renovation projects.

She wants to become the confident mother that she thought she would be, and first needs to re-establish a self-care routine that will encourage her C-section scar to heal. She can then begin to regain her physical fitness, and it will also be important that Jessica is given time to re-engage with her own interests, including pampering herself and socialising.

Initial goals and interventions

1a. Over the next 3 weeks, I will practise a range of activities as Luke's mother, with coaching and reassurance from Kate, the occupational therapist

- Jessica to be supported to spend time with Luke and have skin-to-skin contact
- Jessica to negotiate what baby care support she requires in a 24 hour period (including nappy-changing and bathing), with the support of Kate (OT) and nursery nurses
- Jessica to receive guidance and coaching from Specialist Health Visitors, nursery nurses and Kate regarding infant feeding, to explore future feeding pathways

2a. Over the next 2 weeks I will practice my own self-care, with encouragement and the practical support of Kate and ward staff

- initially, ward staff will provide the physical care of Luke to allow Jessica time for herself to attend to her personal care needs
- Jessica to shower daily with encouragement and prompting from ward staff and Kate
- Jessica will select and sit down to eat lunch on a daily basis with prompting and encouragement form Health Care support staff
- Jessica and Kate will plan and cook a meal together of Jess's selection twice a week

3a. Over the next 3 weeks, I will plan a graded return to physical fitness activities, with advice from Kate and guidance from the physiotherapist

- Jessica to attend the women's health Physiotherapy session with Kate, and discuss appropriate physical activities with physiotherapist
- when medically fit, Jessica, to participate in short walks in the local area with Kate/ward staff

4a. Over the next 2 weeks, I will explore options for continuing an interest, with ideas and assistance from Kate

- Jessica will be encouraged to engage in ward-based activities to explore an activity that is meaningful to her, with guidance from Kate
- Jessica will reflect on activities that she has participated in and identify those which she would like to pursue in the community

Successive goals and interventions

1b. Over the next 2 weeks, I will maintain a routine as Luke's mother, with coaching and reassurance from Kate, the occupational therapist

- Kate and Jessica will write an action plan to help Jess increase her confidence and independence to manage Luke's daily care
- Jessica will receive graded physical support and encouragement from Kate and the ward staff to attend to Luke's daily care needs and eventually to nighttime feeding

2b. Over the next 3 weeks, I will identify strategies to maintain my self-care, with advice and prompts from Kate and ward staff

- Jess to identify the best times for her to attend to her own self-care
- Jess to practise strategies to engage Luke while still attending to her own self-care

3b. Over the next 2 weeks, I will practise a graded return to physical fitness activities, with advice from Kate

- exercise programme to be increased in line with Physiotherapy recommendations
- Kate and the ward staff will accompany Jessica and encourage her to participate in exercise independently

4b. Over the next 3 weeks, I will choose and practise one interest to pursue, with guidance from Kate and practical resources from my family

- Jessica to explore options for pursuing meaningful activities in her local community in preparation for leave and discharge home
- family to bring in chosen resources for Jessica to use while in hospital

Box IV.i   A manager's perspective

As an occupational therapist in a leadership position, I find the formulation process useful as it articulates the unique contribution our therapists have made to the service users' recovery. I can use this information to support the importance of our service and the significant role it has in enabling positive, safe and timely discharges. The occupational therapists using formulations are more confident in describing the value of their interventions to the multi-disciplinary team and all report the format is concise, which results in more time to be with patients rather than writing lengthy documentation.

Box IV.ii   A therapist's perspective

I have found that by using the formulation process it has really helped to give the service user a voice within the wider multi-disciplinary team. It has given me the opportunity to explain what is truly meaningful to the person and help everyone to understand the value of Occupational Therapy interventions within an individual context.

Table IV.i Components of Jessica's occupational identity

Roles/relationships	high school teacher – head of history department; wife, mother, friend and sister
Turning points (inc., changes to physical & social environments)	birth of son 5 weeks ago – birth was long and traumatic, resulting in emergency caesarean section
Interests	running, fell walking, dance – especially Samba – pamper sessions, and home renovation
Volition *(inc., appraisal of ability, expectation of success, values, choices, satisfaction & goals)*	always ambitious with high standards; in a 'happy and stable' relationship; jealous of friend's success and confidence; takes pride in keeping house immaculate; hoped to have children for 4 years and son is much-wanted; hoping to return to work; felt out of control at birth having been excited; self-critical – worries about son, feels hopeless and a failure, but loves son and wants to breast-feed and establish a bond

Table IV.ii Components of Jessica's occupational competence

Routines	worked and engaged in hobbies until just before giving birth – attended Samba group weekly, ran every morning before work, and visited beauty salon regularly; spent many months preparing for baby; now spending most of the day in night clothes; mother looks after baby overnight; husband takes baby for walks and visits his parents when not working; baby feeds for long periods and cries often
Skills	articulate and usually clear about opinions; tires quickly and concentration is affected
Performance	educated to Master's degree level; worked with husband to create beautiful nursery; has stopped attending to own self-care, becomes tearful when baby cries, and is not sleeping well; struggling to lift baby (who is gaining weight as expected) but still capable and able to complete tasks
Environmental contexts	mother is very supportive; husband has adapted to fatherhood well and enjoys tending his baby; baby is being investigated for reflux and milk intolerance; staff are monitoring cleaning of caesarean wound and providing encouragement

References

Baron K, Kielhofner G, Iyenger A, Goldhammer V, Wolenski J (2006) *A User's Manual for the Occupational Self Assessment (OSA) version 2.2*. Chicago: University of Illinois.

Forsyth K, Deshpande S, Kielhofner G, Henrikson C, Haglund L, Olson L, Skinner S, Kulkarni S (2005) *The Occupational Circumstances Assessment Interview and Rating Scale (OCAIRS) version 4.0*. Chicago: University of Illinois.

Parkinson S, Forsyth K, Kielhofner G (2006) *The Model of Human Occupation Screening Tool (MOHOST) version 2.0*. Chicago: University of Illinois.

V Occupational Therapy in an acute mental health service

– an example occupational formulation with measurable goals

Overview

Occupational therapists can make a huge difference in the field of acute mental health, which is all too often a place of occupational deprivation. That said, constructing occupational formulations and measurable goals are undoubtedly challenging in this setting, and it would be impossible for a single occupational therapist to write an occupational formulation for each and every person admitted to an acute psychiatric ward. This is partly because the pace is too fast to allow for enough time to devote to this practice, and partly because some people are sufficiently recovered from a crisis to return home when Occupational Therapy has barely begun. However, the very act of learning to compose an occupational formulation can influence an occupational therapist's professional reasoning and ability to feedback occupational information – even if this is just a verbal account of the summary and the person's key issues.

Mastering the art of writing measurable goals that can be accomplished in a short timeframe might be considered to be even more difficult than composing an occupational formulation when time is limited. How can you focus on a person's life goals when access to their life beyond the ward is so restricted? How can you negotiate realistic timeframes when people are acutely unwell? If these questions have occurred to you, then using the MOHO's taxonomy of occupational engagement (Kilehofner and Forsyth 2008, Pépin 2017) to measure a person's progress towards their goals, may well be a revelation. It can help people work towards their life goals, even within a few days, and certainly within a week or two.

Notice how:

- Danny's preferred pronouns are stated in the introduction
- The occupational therapist accepts the referral with a view to making recommendations that can be followed through after discharge
- The first goal has a timeframe of just 3 days, and the first three goals are all expected to be attained within a fortnight
- Many of the changes in MOHO's taxonomy of engagement, such as *choose, explore, identify, negotiate, plan, practise,* and *re-evaluate* can be made relatively quickly, especially when people are keen to make progress
- A person may explore and practise things within a certain timeframe and therefore achieve the goals that require this, but they can also continue to explore or practise the same issues in subsequent goals. The verbs 'explore' and 'practise' may seem to be less specific than some of the words that therapists ordinarily use to record a person's actions, but they are highly achievable and this makes them incredibly valuable

---

DOI: 10.4324/9781003046301-15

Introduction

Danny is a 27-year-old transgender man (he/him) who took an overdose, intending to die by suicide. During the admission process to an acute mental health unit, Danny asked to be admitted to a male ward, where he was seen automatically by the occupational therapist. An assessment was made of his occupational needs, with a view to making recommendations to be followed through post-discharge.

Occupational assessments completed:

- Occupational Circumstances Assessment Interview and Rating Scale (OCAIRS) (Forsyth et al. 2005)
- informal discussion with Danny and his mother

Occupational identity

Danny was assigned a female identity at birth, and grew up being called Sarah, but 'always' felt that he was a boy and loved climbing, cycling, and being outdoors, as well as drama and playing the trumpet in the school orchestra. He is a single child of Jewish parents and felt loved as a child but also lonely at times, increasingly so as he became more aware of his gender nonconformity, and began to feel disconnected from Jewish culture. Identifying as transgender was affirming in many ways, but also became linked to a sense of stress and shame.

Moving away from home to study Psychology was 'liberating'. Sarah, as he was then, found love with a gay woman, lost her faith, and decided to transition to be a man – beginning hormone therapy before having breast removal surgery when aged 25. By this time, he had split up with his girlfriend and had moved to London to live in shared housing, working mainly in café's and bars as a barista – 'it was easy work and I did it well'.

Danny returned to his hometown last year to help look after his father, who had lung cancer and died 8 months ago. Coming back felt like the right thing to do but was not easy as Danny felt conspicuous when out of the house. He no longer wants to die, but worries about how his mother will manage and feels guilty about being in hospital. Danny wants to find a way to support his mother but is unsure how to do so. And although he does not see himself as returning to Judaism, he misses feeling part of a faith community. Ultimately, Danny wants to 'find happiness again and feel at peace'.

Occupational competence

Danny used to go jogging when in London, and regularly walked in the city parks. He has not spent much time outdoors since returning to his hometown (other than shopping and running errands for his mother), and has not participated in any other interests since university. His mother was more accepting of his transitioning than his father, but it was not much talked about and his mother still worries about what other people in her synagogue may think. She now blames herself for not recognising Danny's distress and is visiting the hospital every day.

At university, Danny belonged to an LGBT+ group and spent time socialising with others. In London, he received support and counselling from the gender identity clinic and did not disclose his gender identity to others. He was apparently accepted as a man by flatmates and colleagues but they did not mix socially, partly because they all worked long unsocial hours in order to afford the rent. Danny now lives rent-free at the family home and has no savings.

When Danny's father became ill, Danny helped with everyday tasks that his mother could not manage such as driving him to appointments and, later, getting him in and out of bed and onto the commode. Danny's mother is now 56. She misses her husband, but is in good health and is a dedicated member of the local synagogue. She is anxious about living alone and yet also wants Danny to be able to get on with his own life and have a fulfilling career.

Key occupational issues

* spending time outdoors
* revising mother/son role
* considering future work options
* finding a sense of community

Summary statement

Danny was studying Psychology at university when he decided to transition. He enjoyed jogging and lived successfully as a man in London, working as a barista.

Since returning home to care for his dying father, Danny feels conspicuous when outside and wants to enjoy being outdoors again. He would like to look after his Jewish mother, who is anxious about living alone but also wants him to have a fulfilling career, and time will be needed to negotiate their relationship and consider future work options. Meanwhile, Danny misses feeling part of a wider community and is keen to address this.

Initial goals and interventions

1. Over the next 3 days, Danny will experience and evaluate time outdoors, facilitated by the occupational therapist (OT)

    * OT to discuss risk issues with the multi-disciplinary team and arrange supervised time outdoors, in the courtyard and in the hospital grounds
    * OT to introduce mindfulness techniques to Danny and discuss the value of being outdoors
    * OT to liaise with Primary nurse to allocate time for Danny to evaluate experiences

2. Over the next fortnight, Danny will plan ideas for a revised mother/son role in negotiation with his mother

- Danny to jot down ideas and set a time to discuss his hopes for the future with his mother

3. Within the next week, Danny will identify supports to help him consider future work options, with direction and information from OT

    - OT to advise re: online careers guidance
    - OT to refer Danny to a Work Matters group at the Recovery College
    - OT to refer Danny to the Individual Placement Support (IPS) team
    - Danny to reflect on skills learned as a barista

4. Over the next month, Danny will explore and choose options for finding a sense of community, with encouragement from OT

    - Danny to investigate LGBT+ forums including Jewish forums and the attitude of other faiths towards LGBT+ people
    - Danny to find out about societies and clubs based on previous interests – cycling, climbing, walking, drama and music

Table V.i Components of Danny's occupational identity

Roles/relationships	single child of Jewish parents; used to be a trumpet player in school orchestra; previously a Psychology student, in gay relationship, a flatmate in shared housing and a barista in café's and bars; recently a carer for father
Turning points (in., changes to physical & social environments)	moving away from home; identifying as transgender; transitioning from Sarah to Danny – beginning hormone therapy and having surgery; father's illness and return to home town; father's death 8 months ago; overdose and hospital admission
Interests	climbing, cycling and being outdoors as well as drama and music
Volition *(inc., appraisal of ability, expectation of success, values, choices, satisfaction & goals)*	always felt he was a boy; lonely at times; felt disconnected from Jewish culture; transgender identity is affirming and leaving home was liberating but still feels stress and shame; found love; lost faith; found work easy and did it well; returning to home town felt like the right thing but also felt conspicuous; no longer wants to die; worries about mother and is unsure how to help her; misses being part of a faith community and wants to find happiness and feel at peace.

Table V.ii Components of Danny's occupational competence

Routines	used to go jogging and walking in city parks; worked long unsocial hours; hasn't spent much time outdoors since returning home, or participated in other interests since university
Skills	it can be inferred that Danny's skills have enabled him to live as a man and find work
Performance	joined LGBT+ group when at university; did not disclose identity to flatmates and colleagues; drove father to appointments and helped with activities of daily living including transfers; shops and runs errands for mother
Environmental contexts	mother more accepting than father – still worries about what others think and blames self for not recognising Danny's distress – and is visiting the hospital every day; she is anxious about living alone but wanting the best for Danny; Danny received counselling from gender identity clinic; is living rent-free and has no savings

Box V.i   A managers' perspective

Occupational formulation is about seeing a person's life as a jigsaw. However the jigsaw pieces are not set in stone, they can be reshaped and a new complete jigsaw can be made.

Formulation enables the person and therapist to deconstruct the jigsaw and examine the pieces, including what may be missing. The uniqueness of occupational formulation is that it enables the person the re-shape the pieces in order to create a new self which functions as a whole more effectively.

Without the acknowledgement of the need for detailed examination of each piece of the jigsaw, and the jigsaw as a whole, there is a risk that a new picture might never be achieved, and thus occupational imbalance would continue.

People often say you need to pick up the pieces – occupational formulation enables you to reshape the pieces and create a new picture.

References

Forsyth K, Deshpande S, Kielhofner G, Henrikson C, Haglund L, Olson L, Skinner S, Kulkarni S (2005) *The Occupational Circumstances Assessment Interview and Rating Scale (OCAIRS) Version 4.0*. Chicago: University of Illinois.

Kielhofner G, Forsyth K, (2008) Occupational engagement: how clients achieve change. In: G Kielhofner ed. *Model of Human Occupation: Theory and Application*. 4th ed. Baltimore: Lippincott, Williams & Wilkins, 101–09.

Pépin G, (2017) Occupational engagement: how clients achieve change. In: RR Taylor ed. *Kielhofner's Model of Human Occupation*. 5th ed. Philadelphia: Wolters Kluwer. 187–94.

VI Occupational Therapy in a primary care service

– an example occupational formulation with measurable goals

Overview

When this formulation was first drafted, the occupational therapist slipped into her customary practice of including a psychological issue, *to improve self-esteem*, among the key issues. Later, the issues were revised to pinpoint the particular *occupations* that were expected to result in improved self-esteem. This is not to say, however, that the inclusion of non-occupational issues can never be justified in a person-centred occupational formulation. For instance, when a person believes that everything hinges on their self-esteem, or is insistent that nothing can be achieved until their alcohol dependency has been addressed, then issues such as self-esteem and alcohol management may make their way into an occupational formulation in order to preserve a therapeutic relationship.

Of course, the best formulations will strengthen a therapeutic relationship by giving a voice to the person's values, interests, and goals. Having earned the person's trust, it should then be easier to assure the person that

- addressing occupational participation is the best way to effect lasting change
- participating in meaningful occupations improves self-esteem, and
- self-care helps us to overcome habits that are less healthy

In other words, psychological issues and intervention-based issues are not separate from a person's occupational issues – they are interrelated – but the unique contribution of an occupational therapist depends on having an occupational focus and on measuring a person's progress in terms of occupational outcomes.

This example shows various ways in which the occupational therapist built rapport: through the use of the Occupational Self Assessment; by structuring the formulation to provide a faithful record of Rebecca's viewpoint; by making use of the first person singular; and by focusing on the person's aspirations.

Introduction

Rebecca is a 25-year-old woman who was diagnosed with anorexia nervosa when aged 14, prior to having Crohn's disease confirmed at the age of 20. She continues to see a range of health practitioners and was referred to Occupational Therapy to assist with her occupational goal attainment.

DOI: 10.4324/9781003046301-16

Notice how:

- The Occupational Self Assessment (Baron et al. 2006) has been used, helping Rebecca to retain a sense of control over her therapy and allowing her to identify the occupations that she values most, as well as those in which she would like to improve her performance
- The first person singular – 'I' – has been used (in this and several other formulations) to enhance the Rebecca's ownership of the goals
- As with many other formulations, Rebecca's Occupational Identity section ends with a focus on her aspirations. Hopes, ambitions, and dreams often go on to form the key issues as this ensures that the associated goals are meaningful, which enhances motivation and adherence. In Rebecca's case, her wish to spend more quality time with her family is included as a key occupational issue

---

Occupational assessments completed:
- Occupational Self Assessment (OSA) (Baron et al. 2006)

Occupational identity

Rebecca enjoyed a range of leisure pursuits during her childhood, such as gymnastics, swimming, and singing in the school choir. At 23, she enrolled in a degree course in nutrition but is now unsure whether she wants to pursue these studies. She sees herself as having always been 'a bit of a perfectionist' and feels that she is mourning for her 'lost self'. She currently wants to reconsider her career options and, following a recent flare-up of her Crohn's symptoms, she has decided to take a yearlong break from her university studies.

Rebecca's rapid weight loss as an adolescent triggered a number of lengthy hospital admissions to a child and adolescent mental health unit, and at this point in her life, Rebecca felt that she had no control over what she could do as she was seen as an anorexic first and a person second. Around this time she also experienced unwanted sexual attention from a former friend and says she responded by trying to make herself unattractive and invisible.

Rebecca visited family abroad last summer and although the experience was stressful she would still like to travel in the future. She values the freedom that living on her own has given her over the past 2 years and also appreciates the support that her parents continue to give her. She frequently experiences guilt and shame for not being as independent as she would like to be, and she looks forward to developing more quality time with her parents and with her younger brother.

Occupational competence

Rebecca comes from a high achieving family and excelled at all subjects at school. Her education was interrupted during her inpatient admissions and yet she still managed to do extremely well in exams. In contrast, her leisure pursuits declined over time. She experiences fatigue and has not had the energy to pursue physical activities for many years, although she has recently started a class in Tai Chi.

Her Crohn's disease has been managed so far without the need for surgery. She is careful about what she eats and is able to cook nutritious meals for herself. Along with ongoing outpatient appointments, she attends a number of private healthcare appointments with a dietician and a psychiatrist. She receives financial support from her parents, and spends time looking after the flat that they bought for her, and investigating possible job opportunities.

While travelling abroad, Rebecca experienced difficulties controlling her diet and lost a considerable amount of weight which she is now gradually regaining. She avoided meeting and socialising with new people and is aware that she has no close friends now. She often tells people that she is fine rather than letting people know how she feels, even when she is experiencing negative thoughts relating to unwanted sexual attention. It seems that her family tends not to discuss emotional issues either. She recognises that developing supportive relationships will be important to her recovery, and comes across as someone who is bubbly and articulate and who relates well to others.

Key occupational issues

- developing new interests
- finding a meaningful primary role
- having quality time with family
- forming valued social relationships

Summary statement

Rebecca is an articulate woman who appreciates her parents' support but also values the freedom of living on her own. She has decided to take a break from her nutrition studies and has recently started a Tai Chi class.

She normally manages her Crohn's disease well, but fatigue has interrupted her pursuit of leisure interests, and she is keen to find a meaningful primary role, to be more independent in the future. Having quality time with her family is also important to her and she would like to form valued social relationships in which she can share her feelings.

Initial goals and interventions

1a. Over the next 4 weeks, I will explore available interests in the local area, with encouragement from the occupational therapist (OT)

- Rebecca to continue attending Tai Chi class
- Rebecca to investigate other options for gentle physical exercise at local sports facilities and evening classes, and options for singing in local choirs
- Rebecca to complete an interest checklist with the OT
- Rebecca to explore options for creative pursuits at home

2a. Over the next 6 weeks, I will re-evaluate options for using a degree in nutrition in a meaningful primary role, in discussion with the occupational therapist

- Rebecca to make an appointment to speak with her personal tutor to discuss future career opportunities

- Rebecca to review reasons for applying to study nutrition and identify strengths and challenges in this field

3a. Over the next 2 weeks I will independently plan options for having quality time with my family

- Rebecca to list interests that she shares with family members and happy times spent with family
- Rebecca to decide which of the options for quality family time would be most feasible

4a. Over the next 8 weeks, I will re-evaluate my experience of friendships and identify the qualities I seek in a valued social relationship, in reflection with the occupational therapist

- Rebecca and OT to discuss Rebecca's needs in a social relationship and identify fears and skills
- OT to discuss stress management techniques and ongoing strategies for managing symptoms of Crohn's

Successive goals and interventions *(in order, as negotiated)*

1b. Over the next 4 weeks, I will choose at least one new interest to pursue with guidance from the occupational therapist

- Rebecca to join local Rock Choir
- Rebecca to continue Tai Chi class and sample a yoga group
- OT to organise silk-painting session with Rebecca

3b. Over the next 2 weeks, I will negotiate planned quality time with my family, with advice from the occupational therapist

- Rebecca to discuss with her mother, the importance of having family time that is not focused on her symptoms
- Rebecca to plan a theatre trip with her parents

3c Over the next 4 weeks, I will practise spending regular quality time with my family, and review my experiences with the occupational therapist

- Rebecca to plan and participate in regular theatre trips, walks and games evenings with family
- Rebecca to plan a walk with her brother

2b. Over the next 6 weeks, I will explore options for a meaningful primary role in the short-term, with direction offered by the occupational therapist

- OT to suggest possible opportunities for voluntary work
- Rebecca to consider options for work experience

1c. Over the next 6 weeks, I will identify the resources required for my chosen interests and sustain my involvement with assistance in problem-solving from the occupational therapist

• Rebecca to research and cost resources for yoga and silk-painting

4b. Over the next 8 weeks, I will review and practise techniques for initiating and managing social relationships with coaching from the occupational therapist

• OT and Rebecca to explore sensory modulation and self-soothing techniques for managing emotions
• OT to train Rebecca in assertion techniques and relaxation techniques
• OT to validate Rebecca's social skills

Table VI.i Components of Rebecca's occupational identity

Roles/relationships	daughter, sister and member of extended family; student of nutrition
Turning points (inc., changes to physical & social environments)	rapid weight loss as an adolescent; diagnosis of anorexia nervosa; hospital admissions; stressful visit to family abroad; unwanted sexual attention; recent flare-up of Crohn's symptoms
Interests	gymnastics, swimming, and singing in a choir
Volition (*inc., appraisal of ability, expectation of success, values, choices, satisfaction & goals*)	unsure regarding whether to pursue studies; wants to reconsider career options and has decided to take yearlong break from studies; always been a bit of a perfectionist; mourning for lost self; felt she had no control – seen as an anorexic first and a person second; tried to make self unattractive and invisible; would like to travel in the future and values freedom of living on own; appreciates support from parents, but experiences guilt and shame for not being as independent as she would like to be; looks forward to developing more quality time with parents and younger brother

Table VI.ii Components of Rebecca's occupational competence

Routines	leisure pursuits have declined over time; recently started Tai Chi; spends time looking after her flat
Skills	appears bubbly, articulate and able to relate to others; experiences fatigue and has no energy for physical activities; has avoided meeting and socialising with new people and has difficulty letting people know how she feels; experiences negative thoughts relating to unwanted sexual attention; recognises the issues that will be important to her recovery
Performance	excelled at school despite interruptions to education; has managed Crohn's without need for surgery; eats and cooks nutritious meals; had difficulty controlling her diet when abroad but is regaining weight now; investigating possible job opportunities
Environmental contexts:	comes from a high achieving family; has ongoing outpatient appointments for Crohn's, and private healthcare appointments with dietician and psychiatrist; receives financial support from parents; family tend not discuss emotional issues and has no close friends now

Box VI.i   A therapist's perspective

The use of occupational formulation has enabled me to regain an occupational focus in a fast-paced mental health clinical role by articulating the occupational issues faced by the people I work with within a short timeframe. The process has assisted me to re-visit people's goals and re-frame their treatment, having re-evaluated where they might consider making changes. I have also been able to take on new referrals with a clearer focus on a person's perception of who they are and how they would like to proceed with their recovery.

The depth of therapeutic alliance created by using this style of formulation has been empowering for me as a clinician but also the people I work with, who have often commented on the process afterwards. Their comments have included: 'you have remembered the words I used to describe this'; 'no-one has asked me these types of questions before'; and 'this sounds just like me – can I share this with my family so they understand?'. The use of this framework has provided an excellent guide to summarise a person's narrative and place this at the forefront of all discussions – a powerful tool in a complex clinical environment.

Reference

Baron K, Kielhofner G, Iyenger A, Goldhammer V, Wolenski J (2006) *A User's Manual for the Occupational Self Assessment (OSA) Version 2.2*. Chicago: University of Illinois.

VII Occupational Therapy in a community mental health service

– an example occupational formulation with measurable goals

Overview

This formulation demonstrates the value of the occupational therapy role in addressing the experience of hoarding, which many believe is likely to be an ever-increasing phenomenon in materialistic societies, where goods are cheap and social connections are hard to maintain. How many of us have friends who have book collections or music collections, or relatives who treasure mementos from their nearest and dearest? How many of us, despite giving so much away to charities, still have a loft full of things that 'might be useful' one day?

There seems to be a natural tendency for people to acquire things and to form an emotional attachment to objects, and occupational therapists have always been interested in the impact that the physical environment has on a person – both good and bad. When collecting and storing objects slip into a pattern of hoarding, a formulation attempts to show how the act of hoarding might have become intricately linked with the person's identity – their values, interests, and habits. It goes on to make a case for key issues that focus on what the person would be able to do if they de-cluttered, rather than focusing on the de-cluttering itself. De-cluttering, disposing of objects, and cleaning might all feature as interventions, but the issues are more personalised and offer a glimpse of a brighter future.

Introduction

Linda is a 60-year-old woman who experiences Seasonal Affective Disorder, has type 2 diabetes, and was admitted to hospital 4 months ago with pneumonia. She is a compulsive hoarder and was referred to the occupational therapist in the Community Mental Health Team to help her to manage her hoarding habits.

Previous attempts to clear Linda's house have been unsuccessful. The occupational therapist has spent time getting to know Linda so that collaborative goals can be established.

Occupational assessments completed:
- Occupational Circumstances Assessment Interview and Ratings Scale (Forsyth et al. 2005)
- Occupational Questionnaire
- Activity Checklist

DOI: 10.4324/9781003046301-17

Notice how:

- the therapist does not reference the non-standardised assessments which have been used: the Occupational Questionnaire (Smith et al. 1986), a diary-based assessment that provides a detailed understanding of a person's routines; and the Activity Checklist published in Recovery Through Activity (Parkinson 2014), which examines preferred activities
- there are themes of loss in Linda's occupational identity, a factor which is often linked to hoarding
- the occupational therapist ensures that positive aspects of Linda's occupational competence are included
- the identity section records Linda's subjective viewpoint and the competence section records objective facts – neither of which are likely to be disputed by Linda
- the key issues utilise Linda's positive motivation
- the initial goals focus on exploring activities, practising tasks and planning ways forward, rather than jumping straight to the ultimate conclusion that Linda will maintain or sustain desired changes
- each goal is linked to a number of actions/interventions

Occupational identity

Linda was a single child and remembers a happy childhood in which she was particularly attached to her mother. Her father worked for the armed forces and she did not like the disruption of moving every few years and of 'never having a home to call our own'. Both parents died when Linda was in her 20s and Linda feels she had to work hard to make a life for herself. Over the years, she enjoyed several close friendships with female friends but they 'married or moved away' and Linda says that she was never interested in male company. She now feels lonely, especially in the winter when it is more difficult to get out and about.

Linda used to love working as an assistant in a pet shop until it closed down 20 or so years ago. She went on to find work in supermarkets and resents losing her last job after having been accused of shoplifting by her employer. That was 15 years ago, at a time when she was sharing her home with half a dozen or more cats. She is upset that they were taken away from her when her house, which she owns, was deemed unfit for habitation 8 years ago. Linda feels ashamed of her property and tries not to interact with her neighbours for fear of what they might think of her. Although she recognises that her house poses a fire risk she believes that she will never be able to stop holding onto things that have a value to her.

She enjoys most crafts – knitting, sewing, and papercraft – as well as baking and 'all things retro'. She is particularly proud of her collection of old sewing machines and she would like to have the space for dress-making again. Recycling is also important to Linda and although she is unsure how she would find the energy, she would like to learn to upholster some of her furniture.

Occupational competence

Linda is well-known in the local charity shops, which she pops into most days, as well as in a nearby café where she has her lunch because her kitchen is currently inaccessible. When she was admitted to the hospital with pneumonia, it was a waitress at the café, called Ann, who realised that Linda was not well and persuaded her to make a doctor's appointment. Ann now visits Linda regularly and tries to help Linda with cleaning. They have cleared a space in Linda's bathroom so that Linda has room for regular strip washes, as personal care was becoming a problem, and Linda pays Ann £5 each week to wash and dry her laundry.

Linda is a caring person who takes an interest in the lives of others – chatting with people she meets out and about. She used to feed stray cats, but has not been doing so for some time – since the back door became inaccessible. Her corridors and other rooms are crammed with craft equipment, furniture, and material for recycling; so much so, that she is unable to see her prized antique sewing machines and is unable to prepare food in her kitchen. Her stairway, however, is mostly clear, as is her bed, and there is no evidence of rodent infestation although the house smells musty.

Linda manages her diabetes medication independently and is not overweight. She tries to look after her mental health by spending as much time as she can out of her house, either shopping, going to car boot sales, or visiting the local parks. It has been a long time since she participated in any crafts, but when she was younger she used to make all her own clothes and soft furnishings.

Key occupational issues

- preparing food in her kitchen
- uncovering and displaying antique sewing machines
- finding a social outlet for craft interests

Summary statement

Linda likes cats, used to love working in a pet shop, and enjoys lots of crafts and 'all things retro'. A friend has helped her to clean her bathroom and she is currently managing her self-care independently. Her kitchen remains inaccessible and Linda misses being able to bake and prepare her own food. She recognises that her home is currently a fire risk and hopes to uncover and display her antique sewing machines. In the meantime, she spends a lot of time out of the house and is interested in finding a social outlet for her craft interests.

Initial goals and interventions

1a. Within the next 3 months, I will have prepared some food (a hot drink and snack) for Ann in my kitchen, with encouragement from Ann and advice from the occupational therapist

- Linda to work with Ann to clean the kitchen, bit by bit, prioritising access to the back door, the sink, fridge, microwave and kettle
- occupational therapist to advise Ann re strategies for de-cluttering, focussing on recycling, and allowing Linda to make decisions

- occupational therapist to refer Linda to the team psychologist to address issues underlying acquisition
- Linda and Ann to investigate help available for 'Hoarders UK' charity

2a. Over the next 6 months, I will choose how to uncover and display my sewing machines, with structured assistance from the occupational therapist

- occupational therapist and Linda to work on one room at a time to uncover sewing machines
- Linda to place objects in 3 bins, to keep forever, to keep for the moment, to give away or recycle
- Linda and occupational therapist to discuss hygiene issues
- occupational therapist to organise the removal of items for recycling
- Linda to organise items to be kept logically and stack or store them safely
- Linda to decide how to display sewing machines

3a. Within 2 months I will have identified a social outlet for my craft interests, with direction from the occupational therapist

- Linda to try out the 'knit and natter group' at the local Social Centre
- Linda to find out about opportunities for upholstery
- Linda to visit the monthly 'Repair Café' at the Community Hub with a view to volunteering her sewing skills to mend users' clothes and soft furnishings
- Linda to consider whether any local outlet might benefit from craft materials and equipment that she is not using.

Box VII.i A therapist's perspective

As an occupational therapist working in a Community Mental Health Service, I often work with individuals who have a range of complex occupational needs, and who also present with a range of additional factors that impact their occupational participation in everyday life. In the context of working in a multidisciplinary setting, I need to be clear about what occupational therapy can deliver, and how we can uniquely use occupation to improve a person's journey by helping each person to lead a fulfilling life. Occupational formulation, following a period of occupational assessment, enables me to make sense of the person's story so far. It helps me to understand the current issues they are facing and, importantly, adds clarity to how we are going to work together and prioritise their occupational goals.

Individuals are often overwhelmed by the issues they face and occupational formulation has provided a structure to enable us to work together to understand and evaluate what is important to them. It has developed my skills by facilitating the engagement process as it communicates that I have understood their story, and individuals often report feeling listened to. Formulation has also developed my ability and confidence to apply MOHO theory to my practice. It supports my thinking by structuring my professional reasoning —making complex scenarios intelligible, and providing a tool that helps individuals to understand how they can work towards change.

Occupational formulation is my bridge in the Occupational Therapy process from assessment to goal setting. It reflects the needs we have identified in Occupational Therapy, and has directly shaped my knowledge of how we can use well-defined goals to make a difference. It has helped me to focus on what to work on, what is most important, and what is most likely to influence occupational change.

In practice, I can often feel constrained by the pace of clinical demands. Clear formulations and goals have supported me to articulate professional involvement in a multi-disciplinary environment with confidence, when a value is often placed on generic styles of working. Although it takes time and commitment in the short-term to embed formulation as part of the Occupational Therapy process, it has developed my skills to be clinically more effective. It encourages me to prioritise the most important aspects of need and plan meaningful goals with the person. Ultimately, this has led to experiences of improved outcomes in therapy.

Table VII.i Components of Linda's occupational identity

Roles/relationships	single child particularly attached to mother; friend; worked as assistant in pet shop and in supermarkets; hoarder
Turning points (inc., changes to physical & social environments)	moved every few years (father was in the armed forces); parents died when in 20s and friends married or moved away; pet shop closed and was accused of shoplifting in last job 15 years ago; house deemed unfit for habitation 8 years ago
Interests	cats, crafts – knitting, sewing & papercraft – baking and 'all things retro'; recycling
Volition *(inc., appraisal of ability, expectation of success, values, choices, satisfaction & goals)*	childhood was happy though disliked disruption of moving; never interested in male company and feels lonely – especially in the winter; upset that cats were taken away from her; feels ashamed of property and fears what neighbours think of her; recognises that house is a fire risk and believes she will never stop holding onto things which have a value to her; recycling is important; proud of collection of old sewing machines; would like to have space for dress-making; unsure how she would find the energy but would like to learn upholstery

Table VII.ii Components of Linda's occupational competence

Routines	pops into charity shops most days; used to feed stray cats but has not done so for some time; spends as much time as possible out of the house, either shopping or at car boot sales or visiting the local parks; hasn't participated in any crafts for a long time
Skills	caring – takes an interest in the lives of others and chats to people she meets; manages diabetes medication independently
Performance	has lunch in a café; personal care was becoming a problem but now has strip washes; collects craft equipment, furniture and material for recycling; used to make all her own clothes and soft furnishings
Environmental contexts	well-known in local charity shops and nearby café; kitchen and back door are inaccessible; waitress from café visits regularly – tries to help with cleaning, has helped to clear space in bathroom, and receives £5 each week to wash and dry laundry; corridors and rooms are crammed but stairway is mostly clear; no evidence of rodent infestation but house smells musty

References

Forsyth K, Deshpande S, Kielhofner G, Henrikson C, Haglund L, Olson L, Skinner S, Kulkarni S (2005) *The Occupational Circumstances Assessment Interview and Rating Scale (OCAIRS) Version 4.0*. Chicago: University of Illinois.

Parkinson S (2014) *Recovery Through Activity: Increasing Participation in Everyday Life*. London: Speechmark Publishing.

Smith NR, Kielhofner G, Watts J (1986) The relationship between volition, activity pattern, and life satisfaction in the elderly. *American Journal of Occupational Therapy*, *40(4)*, 278–83.

VIII Occupational Therapy in a mental health rehabilitation service
– an example occupational formulation with measurable goals

Overview

Here's a formulation with measurable goals depicting a person who appears to have very few interests and who does not demonstrate high levels of volition. She has accessed services for many years and the formulation was developed after she has been in a hospital setting for 6 months. In circumstances like this, occupational therapists are often tempted to restrict the identity section to the person's roles, relationships, interests, and goals in the hospital. Of course, this might be unavoidable if the person has spent most of their life in an institution, but in the vast majority of cases, the richest information concerns their life in the wider society, and it is thankfully very rare for a person's identity to be wholly bound up in their role as a patient. Indeed, the very use of the word 'patient' connotes passivity, whereas the Model of Human Occupation recognises that the role of 'health maintainer' requires active involvement. It is a role that people adopt when they are doing their best to look after themselves in the current circumstances.

Similarly, when a person has spent a period of time in contact with a service, some occupational therapists are tempted to use the competence section to give an account of the person's progress in therapy, including whether or not they have attended certain groups, or even whether or not they are keen to work with the therapist. This pitfall is best avoided, because if a formulation had not been agreed until this point, then the reasons for attending any group might not have been communicated clearly, and the group might not have been relevant to the person's issues. Also, whether or not they are keen to work with the occupational therapist (OT) is irrelevant. It is the therapist's job to engage the client and their volition can be better assessed once the formulation and goals have been agreed.

Introduction

Marcia is a 54-year-old woman who has osteoarthritis in her hips and shoulders. She was diagnosed with Paranoid Schizophrenia in her early 20s and experienced a severe head injury soon afterward. Six months ago, she was involuntarily admitted to a mental health unit and has now been transferred to a rehabilitation ward where Occupational Therapy is an integral part of the service.

DOI: 10.4324/9781003046301-18

Notice how:
- the occupational therapist spent time getting to know Marcia, using a range of occupational assessments, including the Volitional Questionnaire (de las Heras et al. 2007) and the Assessment of Communication and Interaction Skills (Forsyth et al. 1998) to provide a detailed examination of Marcia's relative strengths and limitations
- much of the identity section is focused on Marcia's past roles, before she was admitted to hospital
- even though Marcia does not seem to have any active leisure pursuits, the occupational therapist is able to describe positive interests and preferences and how she likes to spend her time
- the key issues are limited to experiencing *activities*, completing *tasks*, demonstrating a *skill*, and taking *steps* towards self-management, rather than the highest level of doing which involves participating in roles
- the interventions provide step-by-step guidance

Occupational assessments completed:
- Volitional Questionnaire (de las Heras et al. 2007)
- Assessment of Communication and Interaction Skills (Forsyth et al. 1998)
- Model of Human Occupation Screening Tool (Parkinson et al. 2006)
- Interest Checklist and informal conversation
- informal cooking and shopping assessments

Occupational identity

Marcia's parents came to England from Jamaica in the 1950s and Marcia is proud of her Caribbean heritage, enjoying Reggae music as well as Jamaican styling and cooking. She likes bright prints and her favourite food is jerk chicken and rice. She used to enjoy smoking and does not agree with smoking bans, but says it got too difficult to smoke during hospital admissions so she gave it up and does not miss it now.

Marcia 'ran away from home' when she was a teenager and was in a relationship with a man for several years but left him because 'he beat me up'. She is angry that Social Services 'took away my baby' and is distrustful of most contact with services. Over the years, she has lived in hostels and supported housing, and she would like to have a place of her own with a small garden where no-one will bother her.

Marcia does not believe that anything more can be done to manage her joint pain and says that she is too old to work now, but she would have liked to have worked on a flower stall when she was younger. She prefers being in the rehabilitation ward, where it is quieter than the acute ward, and she wishes that she could stay here. She likes to spend her time sitting watching television or sitting in the gardens on a fine day.

Occupational competence

Marcia will often join in song with people who greet her with a Reggae lyric. She declined most occupational therapy interventions in the acute ward but agreed to shop and cook with the rehabilitation occupational therapist to have her favourite food. She was able to walk slowly to the local shop, choose pre-prepared ingredients, and complete the purchase with prompting. In the kitchen, she did not gather or restore objects but was able to handle objects that were brought to her, and contribute to the cooking process with assistance.

Marcia has no contact with any relations, does not always conform to social norms, and argued with fellow residents at her last tenancy. Her speech is not always clear and she is abrupt at times and swears frequently, occasionally apologising for not being 'polite'. She will ask for help with some everyday activities – such as tying her head wrap when the pain in her shoulders is too much. She also benefits from prompts to wash and to brush her teeth, and her skincare and dental care are much improved following the attention she received in the Acute Unit.

Although Marcia does not seek challenges or pursue activities to completion without encouragement, she has clear preferences and shows curiosity. She is more likely to engage with activities in the afternoon, when she will ask questions about the flowers in the garden, and she often spends time watching the chickens from the corridor that runs alongside the chicken coop.

Key occupational issues

* involvement in garden-based activities
* independence in everyday tasks
* developing respectful relationships
* pain management

Summary statement

Marcia is proud of her Caribbean heritage, enjoying Reggae music as well as Jamaican styling and cooking. She also shows an interest in flowers and the unit's chickens, and is being encouraged to get involved with garden-based activities. Eventually, she will need a new tenancy in supported living accommodation where her independence in everyday activities (including self-care, shopping, and cooking) can be supported. In the meantime, the team is encouraging Marcia to show respect for others and they recognise that increased participation will be easier for her if her joint pain can be better managed.

Initial goals and interventions

1. Over the next 6 weeks, Marcia will explore garden-based activities with encouragement from the occupational therapy team

   * gardening instructor to make a point of showing eggs that have been gathered to Marcia, to gauge her response with a view to inviting her to help gather eggs

- OT assistant to bring flowers to Marcia and ask for her opinion, to gauge her response with a view to inviting her to walk around the garden
- all staff to be encouraged to accompany Marcia for short periods of time when she is watching the chickens or sitting in the garden

2. Over the next 12 weeks, Marcia will practise a range of simple everyday tasks with prompts from all staff

   - OT to offer Marcia one-on-one time in the afternoons to practise tasks related to favourite foods
   - OT and nursing staff to work together to prompt Marcia in self-care tasks and provide positive feedback

3. Over the next 8 weeks, the multi-disciplinary team will plan ways to support Marcia to develop respectful relationships

   - OT staff to build rapport with Marcia following the Remotivation Process (de las Heras et al. 2019)
   - staff to thank Marcia when she is polite and model respectful behaviour at all times
   - staff to try to respond to Marcia's requests as soon as possible when she asks politely
   - primary nurse to discuss expectations for politeness at mealtimes with Marcia

4. Over the next 4 weeks, the multi-disciplinary team will identify options for pain management

   - staff to notice if Marcia appears in pain, ask whether she is in pain before initiating any activity, and offer to assist or make adjustments to the activity as necessary
   - OT to ensure that the height of Marcia's bed and bedside chair are appropriate and arrange for a suitable comfy chair to be placed where Marcia can watch the chickens
   - OT to liaise with physiotherapist regarding exercises that Marcia might agree to and initiate discussion of pain management at the next multidisciplinary meeting

---

Box VIII.i   A manager's perspective

After reading the article by Brooks and Parkinson (2018) and attending training on occupational formulation and measurable goals by Sue Parkinson, I felt impelled to instigate these approaches across the mental health service where I work. The BJOT article was disseminated, and internal training workshops were set up for 45 occupational therapists who work across inpatient and outpatient services covering the full lifespan in mental health services. The workshops were led by those of us who had embraced occupational formulation and measurable goals, and our motivation invigorated the remaining sites within the mental health stream to review how they could come on board with this framework.

Time has been the biggest barrier to implementation, as it is for any new skill or programme being commenced, and the use of various professional development forums and supervision has facilitated uptake. As a manager, I have also been in a position to amend our documentation in order to incorporate occupational formulation and measurable goals in our reports, case reviews, and clinical paperwork, which has provided a platform for its ongoing use. Feedback from the workforce has demonstrated that the occupational therapists using occupational formulation have felt a greater connection to their discipline's core philosophy and evidence base – supporting occupational therapists in both discipline-specific and generic roles to place occupation at the forefront of their practice.

Implementation is a longitudinal process and requires a dedicated cycle to embed change, and the most powerful catalyst for change has been the engagement of the stakeholders who will drive the cultural shift. The beauty of occupational formulation is its conceptual underpinnings to the uniqueness of occupational therapy and, therefore, its inherent ability to invigorate a workforce who are eager to return to their discipline-specific roots.

Table VIII.i Components of Marcia's occupational identity

Roles/relationships	parents came to England from Jamaica in the 1950s; previously in a relationship with a man; distrustful of most contact
Turning points (inc., changes to physical & social environments)	ran away from home as a teenager; experienced severe head injury in early 20's; left man because of domestic abuse; services 'took away' baby; lived in hostels and supported housing; involuntarily admitted to acute ward
Interests	likes reggae music, Jamaican styling (bright prints) and cooking (jerk chicken and rice; used to enjoy smoking; watches television and sits in the garden
Volition *(inc., appraisal of ability, expectation of success, values, choices, satisfaction & goals)*	proud of Caribbean heritage; doesn't agree with smoking bans but gave up smoking because of them and doesn't miss it now; angry that services took away baby; would like her own place with small garden where no-one will bother her; doesn't believe anything can be done to manage joint pain; feels too old to work; prefers the rehabilitation ward to the acute ward and wants to stay

Table VIII.ii Components of Marcia's occupational competence

Routines	declined occupational therapy in acute ward; is more likely to engage with activities in the afternoon; often spends time watching the unit's chickens
Skills	able to walk slowly; may not gather or restore objects but is able to handle objects; does not always conform to social norms; speech is not always clear; abrupt at times; swears frequently and occasionally apologises
Performance	argued with fellow residents at her last tenancy; joins in with reggae songs; able to choose pre-prepared ingredients and complete purchases with prompting; contributed to cooking process with assistance; will ask for help with tying her head wrap when pain in shoulders is too much; benefits from prompts to wash and to brush her teeth – skincare and dental care are much improved; does not seek challenges or pursue activities to completion; has clear preferences and shows curiosity; will ask questions about the flowers in the garden
Environmental contexts	no contact with any relations; received support in acute unit with activities of daily living; benefits from encouragement and opportunities to eat favourite food

References

de las Heras CG, Geist R, Kielhofner G, Li Y (2007) *A User's Guide to the Volitional Questionnaire (VQ). Version 4.1.* Chicago: University of Illinois.

de las Heras CG, Llerana V, Kielhofner G [posthumous] (2019) *The Remotivation Process: Progressive Intervention for Individuals with Severe Volitional Challenges: A User's Manual Version 2.0.* Chicago: University of Illinois.

Forsyth K, Salamy M, Simon S, Kielhofner G (1998) *The Assessment of Communication and Interaction Skills (ACIS) Version 4.0.* Chicago: University of Illinois.

Parkinson S, Forsyth K, Kielhofner G (2006) *The Model of Human Occupation Screening Tool (MOHOST) Version 2.0.* Chicago: University of Illinois.

IX Occupational Therapy in a secure mental health service

– an example occupational formulation with measurable goals

Overview

This formulation is one of several in the book where the person has been referred to occupational therapy as part of a 'blanket referral' system. Although this term is commonly understood by health professionals – meaning that someone is automatically referred to a particular service when admitted to a facility, or that the health professional will automatically screen admissions to establish if those admitted require a referral – it is an informal phrase which somehow looks odd in a formal introduction. For this reason, it is recommended that the phrase 'blanket referral' is avoided and that occupational therapists find an alternative way of explaining how they became involved in the person's treatment.

Another tip is to always introduce the person as a woman or a man, or a lady or gentleman, or girl or boy, or by whichever designation the person identifies with, but never as *a* female or *a* male. These latter terms are used frequently by other professions – most commonly in secure services–their use can be dehumanising. Presumably, the terms are abbreviations for a female or a male *patient* or *service user*, and occupational therapists must always acknowledge the uniqueness of each individual, recognising that everyone participates in a number of roles, of which a patient/service user is only one.

Finally, it is usually a good idea, when creating a formulation in a secure service, to mention what the person feels about the circumstances that brought them into hospital, as this is a major turning point, and provides any readers with helpful information as to whether the person regrets their offences or understands why they have been admitted.

Notice how:

- in the introduction, Gary is referred to as a *man*, not a *male*, and use of the term 'blanket referral' has been avoided
- the introduction contains a little more information than usual to alert the reader to known risk factors
- given that Gary is receiving treatment in a long-term setting, there has been time to complete a wide range of assessments – to gain the fullest possible picture – before composing the occupational formulation
- although Gary's feelings regarding his offence are not mentioned explicitly, we learn that he does not like talking of the impact that manic episodes have played in his life, that he feels guilty about his behaviour towards his father, that he does not want to return to his previous lifestyle, and that he hopes to learn skills that will help him to live in the community

---

DOI: 10.4324/9781003046301-19

Introduction

Gary is a 24-year-old man with a diagnosis of Bipolar Disorder. He was diagnosed when he was 18 years old and has required several admissions for inpatient treatment. Whilst experiencing a manic episode, Gary absconded from an Adult Mental Health ward and committed his index offence of a psychotically-driven attack towards his friend. He is currently receiving care in a medium secure psychiatric setting under a Compulsion Order. Gary was referred to Occupational Therapy for assessment.

Occupational assessments completed:

- Model of Human Occupation Screening Tool (Parkinson et al. 2006)
- Occupational Circumstances Assessment Interview and Rating Scale (Forsyth et al. 2005)
- Assessment of Motor and Process Skills (Fisher and Jones 2014)
- Occupational Self Assessment (Baron et al. 2006)
- Interest Checklist

Occupational identity

Gary is passionate about rap music and enjoys spending his time in the ward listening to his favourite rappers and writing his own lyrics. He previously studied music at college and is disappointed that smoking cannabis has impacted on his abilities to complete his studies. Gary would like to return to college to study music in the future and wants to work towards building a career as a rapper.

Gary is frustrated by his current situation and annoyed that he is unable to leave the ward to see his family and friends. Family is very important to Gary, and he feels guilty about his past behaviour towards his father and is happy that they now have a more positive relationship. He worries about his mother who also has a diagnosis of Bipolar Disorder. He is particularly upset that he cannot see his younger brothers, who are 9 and 11, as he does not want them to visit a mental health hospital. He feels isolated from his role within the family and would like to spend time with them outside of the ward.

Gary finds the ward environment stressful and wants some time out of the ward to do the things that he enjoys, such as recording his rap music and seeing his friends. He does not want to return to his previous lifestyle, and hopes that he can get help to build a routine with activities that he enjoys to prevent him from being tempted to smoke cannabis again.

Gary does not like to discuss the times when he has experienced manic episodes and feels angry that mental illness has played such a big role in his life. Gary feels that he has missed out on the opportunities that most teenagers have due to his frequent admissions and is embarrassed that he has not managed to live in the community on his own like the rest of his friends. He is hopeful that by spending longer in the hospital this time, it will give him the chance to learn the necessary skills so that he can stay out of the hospital and live in his own flat independently.

Occupational competence

Despite having a strong interest in music, Gary was previously unable to complete his music studies at college due to missing lectures as a result of smoking too much cannabis. He has remained abstinent from all drugs during his admission and so is hopeful that he will no longer be tempted to abuse substances in the future. Gary is currently engaging with Adult Education sessions within the unit with a focus on completing an open learning course in the music business. During these sessions, he appears focused and is able to retain information well from previous sessions. He has achieved high pass marks during the course and appears realistic when discussing his goal to attend college.

Gary is able to identify a range of interests, however, prior to admission, had limited experience of participating in social and leisure activities due to his previous lifestyle. Within the ward, he is now engaging in various activities, such as learning to play the guitar, arts/crafts, and creative writing. He shows curiosity to try new activities and reports that he is enjoying having a satisfying routine which he would like to sustain on discharge.

Gary's father visits him in the ward weekly and also attends his case reviews to discuss his progress. He is supportive of Gary having time off the ward to spend time with the family, and is understanding of the need to work with staff to ensure that this is timed carefully. He reports that both Gary's mother and brothers are looking forward to seeing him and spending time together as a family.

Gary possesses the skills to complete most activities of daily living, but has had limited opportunities to practise using these activities in the community due to his frequent admissions. He has participated in several cooking and shopping sessions since being admitted this time, and no significant concerns have been identified regarding his functional skills. Gary demonstrates an ability to learn and appears enthusiastic to improve his skills in preparation for future discharge.

Key occupational issues

- enhancing role within the family
- going to college to study music
- developing skills to manage independent living

Summary statement

Gary is passionate about rap music and is motivated to progress his studies so that he can develop a career in the music industry. Family is very important to Gary and he values the support he receives from his father. He looks forward to being able to spend time with his family off the ward in the future. Gary has had limited experience in managing household tasks, but demonstrates basic skills in his activities of daily living and shows an ability to learn. He would like to develop his skills and would like to live independently in his own flat.

Initial goals and interventions

1a. Over the next month, Gary will identify how to enhance his role within his family, with encouragement and suggestions from his occupational therapist

- Gary to plan how to make the best use of his time with his father when he visits the ward
- Gary to send a card to his mother
- Gary to talk with others about how to maintain his relationship with his younger siblings

2a. Over the next 2 months, Gary will explore options for studying music at college, with guidance from his occupational therapist

- Gary and the occupational therapist to review college websites to identify appropriate courses
- Gary to attend the ward music group to develop his leadership skills
- Gary to keep a record of his musical achievements

3a. Over the next 3 months, Gary will practise a range of skills necessary for independent living, with coaching and structure from the occupational therapy team

- Gary to attend weekly cooking sessions
- Gary to continue to take responsibility for tidying and cleaning his bed area, and managing own laundry
- occupational therapist to assess Gary's financial management skills

Box IX.i A therapist's perspective

Within my practice as an occupational therapist, I had the opportunity to develop skills using a range of standardised assessments and was confident in my abilities to conduct these with patients in order to gather quality Occupational Therapy assessment. I was, however, becoming increasingly frustrated regarding my abilities to translate the information gained from assessments into appropriate goals with patients. I found the goal-setting process to be challenging and therefore time-consuming.

Since being introduced to the occupational formulation process, my practice has changed significantly. I realised that previously I did not dedicate time to consider all of the assessment information and instead was attempting to move very quickly from the assessment stage to delivering treatment plans. Although I had thought that the goals were client-centred, key information was being missed.

I have particularly enjoyed considering a patient's occupational identity, as it has encouraged me to spend time considering the person's narrative, and it ensures that I have captured what really matters to them. This has been beneficial when building therapeutic rapport with patients, and I feel that when using this process I really get to know my patients well. It has also meant that patients who had previously been reluctant to engage in Occupational Therapy are now able to see the purpose of sessions more clearly and are therefore more interested to participate in sessions. Documenting information regarding the patient's occupational identity has also been helpful when attending meetings with other professionals as I am able to feedback information that may have been missed before.

Once I have identified the key occupational issues, I have found that translating these into measurable goals has been straightforward and easy to negotiate with patients. It has meant that I am confident that goals are truly patient-centred and are addressing the specific issues that the patient wishes to work on. It has also meant t hat I am able to clearly communicate the purpose of interventions to other professionals and highlight the benefit of Occupational Therapy, which helps to promote my role within the team.

Table IX.i Components of Gary's occupational identity

Roles/relationships	previously a music student; has improved relationship with father; mother also has Bipolar Disorder and has two younger brothers (aged 9 and 11)
Turning points (inc., changes to physical & social environments)	diagnosis of bipolar Disorder aged 18; did not complete studies; attacked a friend when manic; detained in medium secure unit
Interests	rap music (including recording own music); seeing friends
Volition (*inc., appraisal of ability, expectation of success, values, choices, satisfaction & goals*)	enjoys listening to favourite rappers and writing own lyrics; disappointed that smoking cannabis impacted on college studies and would like to return to college; wants a career as a rapper; is frustrated by ward restrictions. family is very important; feels guilty about his past behaviour happy to have a more positive relationship with his father; worries about his mother and does not want brothers to visit a secure hospital; feels isolated from family and wants to spend time off the ward as it is stressful; does not want to return to previous lifestyle; angry re impact of mental illness and missing out on things; embarrassed about not having managed to live on his own; hopes to learn skills and live in own flat

Table IX.ii Components of Gary's occupational competence

Routines	limited experience of participating in social and leisure activities prior to admission; now engaging in a satisfying routine; father visits weekly
Skills	appears focused and able to retain information from previous education sessions; no evident problems with skills
Performance	previously missed lectures when smoking cannabis; now abstinent from all drugs; has started open learning course in music business, achieving high pass marks; shows curiosity to try new activities; has demonstrated basic cooking and shopping abilities; appears enthusiastic to improve skills
Environmental contexts	accesses Adult Education sessions, guitar lessons, arts/crafts, and creative writing sessions, cooking and shopping sessions; lacks opportunities to practise community skills; father is supportive and attending case reviews; mother and brothers look forward to seeing him

References

Baron K, Kielhofner G, Iyenger A, Goldhammer V, Wolenski J (2006) *A User's Manual for the Occupational Self Assessment (OSA) version 2.2*. Chicago: University of Illinois.

Fisher AG, Jones KB (2014) *Assessment of Motor and Process Skills. Vol 2: User Manual.* 8th ed. Fort Collins, CO: Three Stars Press.

Forsyth K, Deshpande S, Kielhofner G, Henrikson C, Haglund L, Olson L, Skinner S, Kulkarni S (2005) *The Occupational Circumstances Assessment Interview and Rating Scale (OCAIRS) version 4.0*. Chicago: University of Illinois.

Parkinson S, Forsyth K, Kielhofner G (2006) *The Model of Human Occupation Screening Tool (MOHOST) version 2.0*. Chicago: University of Illinois.

X   Occupational Therapy in a prison service

– an example occupational formulation with measurable goals

Overview

Formulations in prison services give occupational therapists a much-needed opportunity to build rapport, by demonstrating their understanding of what people have been through and where they have come from. More than this, the allow occupational therapists to share prisoners' strengths with the team – building positivity through an appreciation of the strengths that exist and can be built on. Thereafter, they lead to finely graded goals, which enable everyone to see the progress being made towards the things that are really important to the individuals concerned, and that will benefit them in their lives beyond the prison; whether they are released in a matter of months, or years, or decades.

This formulation also shows how a simple version of Goal Attainment Scoring (GAS) (Turner-Stokes 2009) may be used to measure the person's progress. Arran's goal attainment is given a score of 0 if he meets the goal as expected – making the stated level of change within the stated timeframe and with the stated level of support. If, for some reason, he does not make any progress, the score of -1 is given, and were he to go backwards, a score of –2 could be given. The system also allows an extra point (+1) to be awarded if Arran meets the goal as expected but also makes more changes, *or* makes the change in a shorter timeframe *or* with less support than expected. Finally, a score of +2 can be given if Arran exceeds expectations with regards to two or more of these elements: the level of change, the timeframe, or the level of support. Ideally, if the goals have been set to provide the right level of challenge, he will score an average of nought overall.

Introduction

Arran is a 38-year-old man serving a life sentence for murder and has served 9 years to date. Arran can now begin the process of progression through the prison system in preparation for release; however, substance misuse is a significant barrier limiting progression. Arran was referred to Occupational Therapy by Forensic Psychology after he highlighted a concern over his ability to complete everyday activities expected for life outside prison.

Occupational assessments completed:
*   Occupational Circumstances and Interview Rating Scale (OCAIRS) (Forsyth *et al.* 2005)
*   Assessment of Motor and Process Skill (AMPS) (Fisher and Jones 2014)

DOI: 10.4324/9781003046301-110

Notice how:

- Arran's feelings regarding his offence have been noted – 'I shouldn't have done what I did, but I just couldn't manage'
- the Assessment of Motor and Process Skills (AMPS) (Fisher and Jones 2014) provides the occupational therapist with detailed evidence of transferable skills – he is 'quick to notice what needs to be done and find solutions', 'paces himself', and 'demonstrates good strength and effort'
- starting the summary with positives about Arran's life is even more important, if the therapist is to be an effective advocate for a prisoner in a system which struggles to balance rehabilitation with punishment
- issues that extend beyond release from prison can be agreed, even though Arran is serving a life sentence because they can be graded in terms of the occupational changes that Arran makes towards their eventual resolution
- Arran's average goal attainment so far is nought, showing that he is meeting goals as expected

Occupational identity

Arran is a father, grandfather, and son, and would like to be more involved in his family. He has employment in the prison cleaning party, and wants to be employed and to help his mum after release. These roles have proved important to Arran, not only providing structure, a sense of productivity, and a focus, but also in helping him manage his mental wellbeing – 'it helps me feel better about myself'.

When Arran was younger, he could not wait to leave home. He obtained a council flat of his own for a few months and soon experienced difficulties coping due to substance misuse and anti-social behaviours. He also worked for a few days at a fish factory in his local area and regrets that his lifestyle 'got in the way' and he lost this job. His first prison sentence was when he was 16 years old and he had multiple short term sentences prior to his life sentence – 'I shouldn't have done what I did, but I just couldn't manage'.

Arran's current pastimes include cleaning, scrabble, and jigsaws – activities which he says are more a result of them being readily available rather than being of interest. He sometimes feels old before his time and misses the times when he had the energy to play football and go to the gym regularly.

Arran feels that becoming older in prison and losing his father and his brother has provided him with the motivation to turn his life around. He feels worried he will not manage life outside and is unsure about whether he will be able to succeed. He feels a sense of unworthiness given his offence and is unsure what a typical life for a 38-year-old would look like, but wants to get a better control over his substance use and establish a meaningful and positive life beyond prison.

Occupational competance

Arran fulfils the role of father (to a daughter), son, and grandfather (to a 3-year-old grandson) as well as he could, given the prison restrictions and limitations: seeing his family at visits as well as having daily phone calls and exchanging frequent letters. He also manages personal and domestic activities in prison very well and is hugely competent in his work role which involves undertaking general cleaning roles in the prison as well as specialist biohazard cleaning jobs. Arran is commended by staff for his commitment to this role, in which he has sustained involvement despite intermittent substance use and numerous challenging personal stressors, including breaking up with the mother of his son, and the death of his father and brother.

Although Arran is competent in his prison-based roles, he lacks experience and knowledge of the everyday activities that would be expected of him after release and for the process of progression. This includes money management, cooking, structuring his free time, managing a work role without the support the prison environment affords, and managing a tenancy. Previously, at times when he has felt hopeless, he has disengaged from the multi-disciplinary team and found ways to use drugs.

Occupational therapy assessment has shown that Arran has the motor and process skills that would be necessary for independence in daily activities as he is quick to notice what needs to be done and find solutions. He still struggles to get up in the morning and has not played football or gone to the gym for over a year, but paces himself when working and demonstrates good strength and effort.

Key occupational issues

- maximising family involvement
- obtaining future work
- practising everyday activities
- finding energy for active leisure interests

Summary statement

Arran enjoys contact with his mother, daughter, and young grandson through daily phone calls and frequent letters, and he values his work in the prison cleaning party. He would like to be more involved with his family and help his mum after release. This would be helped by obtaining future work, most likely in the cleaning sector where Arran has proven competencies. He is less sure about managing everyday activities required for independent living and would benefit from time to practise money management and cooking. He would also like to feel young again and find the energy for active leisure interests.

Initial goals and interventions

1a. Over the next 3 weeks, Arran will plan ways to maximise his family involvement while still in prison, with guidance from the occupational therapist (OT)

- Arran to ask family members what they appreciate most in terms of contact
- Arran to plan phone calls that demonstrate an interest in his family
- Arran to write letters that give family members positive feedback

Goal Attainment Scoring: **0**

2a. Over the next 4 weeks, Arran will investigate the steps needed to obtain future work with advice and supervision from the occupational therapist

- OT & Arran to list the steps to consider for employment and review gaps in Arran's' experience
- OT to review Arran's CV and interview skills
- Arran to receive a written appraisal of his work in the cleaning party
- identify the things which require further research/questions answered and explore how this information can be sought

Goal Attainment Scoring: **0**

3a. Within 2 weeks, Arran will have identified his strengths and limitations with regard to everyday activities, with structure and feedback from the occupational therapist

- Arran to complete Occupational Self Assessment (Baron et al. 2006)
- OT and Arran to discuss strengths and limitations
- OT to provide positive feedback

Goal Attainment Scoring: **0**

4a. Within 1 week, Arran will have explored and identified some active leisure interests which could be tried in prison with guidance from the OT

- Arran to complete interest checklist

Goal Attainment Scoring: **0**

1b. Over the next 6 weeks, Arran to maintain family involvement while in prison, with encouragement from the occupational therapist

- Arran to plan topics to discuss at family visit

Goal Attainment Scoring: **0**

2b. Over the next 8 weeks, Arran to practise skills required for obtaining future work and explore future work options with advice and information from the occupational therapist

- Arran to continue working in the prison cleaning party and discuss the possibility of increased challenges
- OT and Arran to research the feasibility of working in biohazard cleaning, given his convictions

Goal Attainment Scoring: **−1**

3b. Over the next 8 weeks, Arran will practise a range of relevant everyday activities, facilitated by the occupational therapist and prison services

- OT to liaise with officers & education service to discuss skills to be developed/ approaches to be used
- Arran to meet with the life skills officers and education service to plan involvement in everyday activities
- OT to monitor and obtain feedback

Goal Attainment Scoring: **+1**

4b. Within 2 weeks, Arran will have explored ways to try out potential interests in prison, in collaboration with the occupational therapist

- OT to arrange taster sessions of identified interests

- OT to liaise with prison officers to negotiate access

Goal Attainment Scoring: **0**

Table X.i Components of Arran's occupational identity

Roles/relationships	father, grandfather and son; works in prison cleaning party; once worked for a few days in a fish factory
Turning points (inc., changes to physical & social environments)	living on own as a teenager; misusing substances; multiple short-term prison sentences; life sentence for murder; brother and father dying; finding structure and focus in prison work
Interests	previously interested in football and going to the gym; interests now limited and include cleaning, scrabble and jigsaws
Volition *(inc., appraisal of ability, expectation of success, values, choices, satisfaction & goals)*	could not wait to leave home when young; regrets past behaviours – 'I just could not manage'; would like to be more involved in his family; wants employment and to help his mum after release; work helps him to feel better about himself; feels old before his time and misses having more energy; motivated to turn life around; worried he will not manage life outside; feels a sense of unworthiness; unsure what a typical life for a 38-year-old is; wants better control over substance use and a meaningful/positive life beyond prison

Table X.ii Components of Arran's occupational competence

Routines	sees his family at visits – has daily phone calls with them and exchanges frequent letters; has sustained involvement in work role despite intermittent substance use; struggles to get up in the morning; hasn't played football or gone to the gym for over a year
Skills	has motor and process skills necessary for independence – quick to notice what needs to be done and find solutions, paces self when working, and demonstrates good strength and effort
Performance	fulfils the role of father (to a daughter), son and grandfather (to a 3-year-old grandson) as well as he can, given prison restrictions and limitations; manages personal and domestic activities in prison very well and is hugely competent in his work role; has coped with numerous personal stressors (break-up of relationship and bereavements); lacks experience and knowledge of everyday activities such as money management, cooking, structuring his free time, managing a work role without the support the prison environment affords, and managing a tenancy
Environmental contexts	undertakes general cleaning roles in the prison as well as specialist biohazard cleaning jobs; commended by staff for his commitment in work role

Box X   A therapist's perspective

From a service user viewpoint, individuals have said they have felt involved and played an active part in designing their therapy, as the process of occupational formulation has facilitated personally meaningful, client-centred goals and enabled co-production. Identifying areas of change, translating these into goals and agreeing interventions in collaboration with the person has increased service user engagement and improved an understanding of the Occupational Therapy focus. More than this, the use of goal attainment has built motivation, determination, and personal causation – often proving to be a therapeutic intervention in itself.

As a therapist, the use of the case formulation – and the formula presented for goal setting particularly – has ensured I maintain an emphasis on occupational participation and occupational change, which has positively influenced job satisfaction. Treatment outcomes have been easier to extract – allowing occupational change to be evidenced and its impact and relevance to wider service aims to be articulated. Surprisingly, occupational formulation has also been useful in teasing out when an occupational approach is not the appropriate approach to assist a person to move forward. The rationale can then be clearly and robustly articulated to the team.

References

Baron K, Kielhofner G, Iyenger A, Goldhammer V, Wolenski J (2006) *A User's Manual for the Occupational Self Assessment (OSA), Version 2.2*. Chicago: University of Illinois.

Fisher AG, Jones KB (2014) *Assessment of Motor and Process Skills. Vol 2: User manual* (8th ed.) Fort Collins, CO: Three Stars Press.

Forsyth K, Deshpande S, Kielhofner G, Henrikson C, Haglund L, Olson L, Skinner S, Kulkarni S (2005) *The Occupational Circumstances Assessment Interview and Rating Scale (OCAIRS) Version 4.0*. Chicago: University of Illinois.

Turner-Stokes L (2009) Goal attainment scaling (GAS) in rehabilitation: a practical guide. *Clinical Rehabilitation, 23*, 362–70. DOI: 10.1177/0269215508101742.

XI Occupational Therapy in a service for homeless people

– an example occupational formulation with measurable goals

Overview

This formulation represents some of the fabulous work that occupational therapists do with people who are experiencing homelessness. Brian is currently staying in a hostel, which undoubtedly makes it easier for the occupational therapist to negotiate occupational goals, but occupational formulations can still be pivotal when people are rough-sleeping. In such cases, the therapist would still need to listen to each person's story in order to understand the complexity of their unmet needs, and a well-constructed formulation could prove invaluable when advocating for their rights and helping them to access the services that they require.

Many people who live in precarious circumstances and who experience long-standing mental health problems end up having treatment plans which state what the team is going to do – e.g., monitoring the person's health and arranging for accommodation. Plans may also be produced which focus on ideas about what the person should stop doing (e.g., restricting alcohol intake), or which focus on standards and targets that the person is expected to follow (e.g., attending certain appointments and taking medication). How refreshing, to see a focus on the issues that are meaningful for Brian. Brian has even agreed to include self-care as an issue, despite feeling that he can manage independently, because the occupational therapist suggested that he would benefit from '*maintaining*' mental health and self-care. This provides the occupational therapist with an opening to review Brian's alcohol intake, without (quite literally) making an issue out of this.

Introduction

Brian is a 39-year-old man who was recently discharged from hospital following a 12-month admission, during which he was diagnosed with Paranoid Schizophrenia. He has a history of binge-drinking and is currently staying in a hostel for homeless people. He was referred to an occupational therapist at the mental health day service to support his occupational needs.

Occupational assessments completed:
- Occupational Circumstances and Interview Rating Scale (OCAIRS) (Forsyth et al. 2005)
- Assessment of Motor and Process Skills (Fisher and Jones 2014)
- Model of Human Occupation Screening Tool (Parkinson et al. 2006)

DOI: 10.4324/9781003046301-111

> **Notice how:**
>
> - the occupational therapist has used the Occupational Circumstances and Interview Rating Scale (OCAIRS) (Forsyth et al. 2005) to gain a full picture of Brain's past and present roles, routines, and interests
> - Brian's resourcefulness and his ability to survive are acknowledged, as well as the difficulties he has faced
> - when analysing the components of Brian's Occupational Competence, one can appreciate the detail in which the occupational therapist understands his current routine
>
> Brian's second goal is to *re-evaluate* his skills for maintaining good mental health and self-care. Although re-evaluation often comes later on in a series of goals – after a period of practising something, for instance – it makes sense to start with re-evaluation for Brian, before any clearer goals can be agreed

Occupational identity

Brian is unsure what his diagnosis means and is glad to be out of the hospital and to have a secure place to live. He used to take pleasure in living in a flat on his own, but prior to being in the hospital, he had been evicted due to rent arrears and was rough-sleeping in a tent. This was a traumatic period of his life that he describes as 'tough' due to being cold and hungry. He felt excluded and stigmatised, but held on to the need to survive and remembers good things too, including the freedom he had and the kindness of strangers. Eventually, however, he says he deliberately got arrested for shoplifting in order to access support. Since moving to the hostel, he feels that he can manage his personal self-care, but feels that the future is out of his control and finds it hard to see how he can make any changes.

He left his family home when he was 18 because his Dad had died and he was not getting on with his mother. He is pleased to have phone contact with her again, but has no other expectations regarding their relationship and does not anticipate getting back in touch with his brother or with any previous contacts that he had as a young man.

After leaving school, Brian worked as a labourer on construction sites and drove a pick-up truck. He enjoyed drinking with his workmates after work and was proud to be earning good money – enough to go to rock concerts. These days, he feels tired most of the time and although he would like to work again and has an interest in driving and gardening, he cannot imagine finding work in the future. He still enjoys music and recounting past concerts, and he is also interested in religion and describes himself as an animal lover. More than anything, he wants to get his own place to live.

Occupational competence

Brian survived sleeping rough for almost 2 years prior to his admission and is now living in a hostel in the city centre, in a studio-type flat. He has an ensuite bathroom and basic kitchen facilities, as well as access to a communal outdoor space. There are also communal laundry facilities and a dining room where cooked meals are prepared that have to be purchased. Brian is taking his medication independently and, although his self-care fluctuates at times, he has proved to have good money management skills – successfully budgeting his money to pay for his rent and food. He also budgets for beer – (he drinks four cans of beer every evening and does not smoke).

Brian's mother still phones once a month. Other than this, Brian keeps himself to himself in the hostel and the day service setting unless approached by workers, who are the only people to visit him in his room. At the day service, he has participated in gardening tasks with encouragement from the occupational therapist, and clearly has good motor and process skills. He also has good conversation skills on a one-to-one level. When in a group setting, he tends to stay quiet or use non-verbal skills to communicate his opinions.

Brian follows the same daily routine: breakfasting in the dining room before leaving the hostel to pray on his own at the local Catholic Church, and then walking for 30 minutes to the Day Service and spending 3-4 hours there, where a midday meal is provided. He then walks back to the hostel, buying beer on the way, and spends the evening in his room drinking and watching television. The only changes to this routine are when he leaves the day service early once a week to collect his benefits, and when the Day Service is closed on a Sunday, and he goes to the park to feed the birds and cats, and buys chips for his tea from a fish and chip shop.

Key occupational issues

- having own place to live
- maintaining mental health and self-care
- using interests to gain work
- establishing a support network

Summary statement

Brian is a resourceful man, who describes himself as an animal lover and has an interest in religion. Having previously slept rough, he would love to have a place of his own, and meanwhile, he is taking steps to look after his mental health and his self-care. Although he feels that his future is out of his control, he clearly has skills to offer and would like to work again, perhaps using his interests in driving, gardening, or tending to animals. In the meantime he would benefit from expanding his support networks, starting by developing connections at the church he attends.

Initial goals and interventions

1a. Over the next 2 months, I will identify a plan for having my own place to live and practise relevant skills, in collaboration with the occupational therapist (OT)

- explore my values regarding what is important for having my own place
- meet the OT in my current flat and start to gather personal possessions that will support the transition into my own place
- identify my strengths and the skills I will need for looking after my own place
- attend the Practical Living Skills group to practice skills and review my knowledge related to home management, e.g., the rights and responsibilities of being a tenant
- adapt my routine to support graded use of my current kitchen facilities

2a. Over the next month, I will re-evaluate the skills needed to maintain my mental health and self-care, with encouragement and coaching from the occupational therapist and the wider team

- identify what I do on a daily basis to keep me well, in terms of a healthy lifestyle (including review of alcohol use)
- work with the OT to produce a Wellness Recovery Action Plan with a practical focus
- adapt my routine to build in alternative evening activities – budgeting to get materials for a hobby that can be done in my own flat, perhaps connected to an interest in music
- join a gym group with the support of the OT Assistant (OTA) initially

3a. Over the next 4 months, I will explore future work options, based on my interests, with advice and direction from the occupational therapist

- increase attendance in work style groups e.g., gardening in day service to build endurance, concentration span and confidence
- set objectives with the OT to increase communication and interaction within these groups
- explore options for participating in a volunteer gardening scheme
- attend open days of supported employment

4a. Over the next 3 months, I will plan how to build a support network, with ideas and structured involvement occupational therapist

- explore meaningful interests and try out activities with, support of OT/ OTA e.g., computers, football
- focus on building social skills
- visit church to source information about church-related activities and get ideas about how I can become more involved
- arrange to meet with priest/parish warden (with OT if permission gained)
- plan to attend one church event (outside of usual individual visits to church)

Box XI.i   A therapist's perspective

What I really like about this occupational formulation is how it captures the person and keeps occupation central. Over a period of time, the experience of homelessness and housing instability can dominate a person's time use and routines, as well as influencing their everyday activities. This has the potential to create the role of 'homeless service user', which can be all-consuming – focused on resourcefulness and the presenting challenges. However, exploring a person's occupational influences has the power to bring other interests, roles, and values to the fore, to help extend a person's story beyond homelessness and guide meaningful goals for intervention.

The structure of an occupational formulation helps maintain an occupational perspective. As occupational therapy within homelessness is a growing area of practice, keeping occupation central is critical. It demonstrates our unique and important contribution to improving the lives of people who experience homelessness.

Table XI.i Components of Brian's occupational identity

Roles/relationships	Dad died and did not get on with mother; has re-established contact with her, but lost contact with brother, friends, and workmates; has previously worked as a labourer and pick-up truck driver
Turning points (inc., changes to physical & social environments)	Left family home at 18; glad to be out of the hospital and have a secure place to live; was evicted due to rent arrears and was rough-sleeping in a tent; got arrested for shoplifting to access support
Interests	Music and recounting past rock concerts, driving and gardening, religion and animals
Volition *(inc., appraisal of ability, expectation of success, values, choices, satisfaction & goals)*	Unsure what diagnosis means; used to enjoy living in own flat; eviction and rough-sleeping were traumatic – felt excluded and stigmatised, but held on to need to survive; remembers good things including freedom and kindness of strangers; feels that he can manage personal self-care, but feels future is out of his control and finds it hard to see how he can make changes; pleased to have phone contact with mother but no expectations of this relationship; used to enjoy drinking with workmates and was proud to earn good money; feels tired most of the time; would like to work but cannot imagine finding future work; wants own place to live

Table XI.ii Components of Brian's occupational competence

Routines	Slept rough for almost 2 years; does not smoke but drinks four beers every evening; mother phones once a month; leaves the hostel after breakfast to pray at local church, walks 30 minutes to Day Service, spends 3-4 hours there, walks back to hostel, buys beer, spends evenings watching TV; collects benefits once a week; feeds birds and cats in a park on Sunday, and buys chips for his tea
Skills	Good motor and process skills; good 1:1 conversation skills; quiet in group settings – communicating opinions non-verbally
Performance	Survived sleeping rough; is taking medication independently but self-care fluctuates; has good money management skills – successfully budgeting money to pay for rent, food and beer; keeps self to himself in the hostel and day service setting unless approached by workers
Environmental contexts	Currently living in a city centre hostel – in a studio-type flat with ensuite bathroom and basic kitchen facilities, access to communal outdoor space, communal laundry facilities and a dining room where cooked meals are prepared and sold; accesses Catholic church and Day Services, and receives benefits; workers, are the only people who visit him in his room

References

Fisher AG, Jones KB (2014) *Assessment of Motor and Process Skills. Vol 2: User Manual.* 8th ed. Fort Collins, CO: Three Stars Press.

Forsyth K, Deshpande S, Kielhofner G, Henrikson C, Haglund L, Olson L, Skinner S, Kulkarni S (2005) *The Occupational Circumstances Assessment Interview and Rating Scale (OCAIRS) Version 4.0.* Chicago: University of Illinois.

Parkinson S, Forsyth K, Kielhofner G (2006) *The Model of Human Occupation Screening Tool (MOHOST) Version 2.0.* Chicago: University of Illinois.

XII Occupational Therapy in a traumatic stress service

– an example occupational formulation with measurable goals

Overview

There are times when you really need to think very carefully about the balance of positives and negatives in a formulation, and this is a case in point. Banita is seeking asylum and her history is filled with distressing circumstances, and the occupational therapist has been able to start and end the Identity section with positives. Otherwise, however, Banita's experiences of being rejected and abused, and her feelings of shame, fear, and isolation are faithfully reported. To do otherwise, would risk misrepresenting her story and suggest that the therapist either did not understand Banita's history, or lacked sufficient empathy.

Remember that if you have no reason to disbelieve a person, there is no need to interrupt the narrative flow with words such as 'apparently', or phrases such as, 'she states that …', or 'she reports that …'. The Identity section should try to provide an authentic account of the person's subjective viewpoint and although you have the right to decide whether it would be wise to distinguish between opinion and fact, it is best to think twice before tampering with the person's story.

Finally, although integration is a common problem that affects most people seeking asylum, the occupational therapist chooses plain English – 'getting to know people' – to describe the issue. If you avoid the use of standard phrases and always choose the same words that you used with the person themselves, it helps to keep the issues person-centred and relevant to the individual.

Notice how:

- Banita was able to use the Occupational Self Assessment (OSA) (Baron et al. 2006) with the help of an interpreter
- when analysing the components of Banita's Occupational Identity, it is apparent that numerous life turning points have shaped her life story
- in the Competence section, the occupational therapist takes care to explain aspects of the asylum process that readers might not otherwise understand, e.g., the restrictions of the payment card system
- the occupational therapist picks out phrases that have already been used in the preceding Identity and Competence sections to define the issues: getting to know people, expressing true self, and developing skills
- the formulation and goals are followed by a record of the achievements that Banita makes over a 3 month period

---

DOI: 10.4324/9781003046301-112

Introduction

Banita is a 27-year-old woman who entered the UK using a false passport and is now seeking asylum. She has been placed in the North East of England while her claim is examined, and was referred to Occupational Therapy in a Traumatic Stress service after presenting with low mood and suicidal ideation.

Occupational assessment completed:

* Occupational Self Assessment (Baron et al. 2006) translated into Urdu via an interpreter

Occupational identity

Banita had a comfortable childhood in India and enjoyed art and dancing. There were no notable issues until her teens, when she fell in love with a young man from a different caste. Her family had wanted her to enter an arranged marriage and she was shunned by them. Her sadness at being rejected was mixed with the shame that she had brought dishonour on her family, and fears for her own life. Her mother told her that she must never see any of them again as she 'did not want her brothers to dirty their hands with her blood'.

She married and moved away with her husband, and they were happy in the beginning, but Banita soon felt inadequate and afraid. Her mother-in-law, who lived with them, started to criticise her housework and cooking, and became verbally abusive – telling Banita that she was worthless. Banita worked in the house 'like a slave', and when she did not become pregnant she was told that she must be a bad person. She was raped and beaten by her husband – sometimes leading to hospital visits – and Banita felt trapped and alone for many years.

Fourteen months ago, Banita took a passport belonging to a sister-in-law, and escaped her marital home with the help of her auntie who gave her money so she could fly to the UK. Banita was frightened about travelling on her own without having a clear destination, but could not think what else to do. She now lives in a house with three other women, none of whom share a common language, and feels isolated and hopeless about her situation as her asylum claim has recently been refused.

Banita feels self-conscious when using the asylum seekers' payment card when paying for necessities, and is afraid of drawing attention to herself in the supermarket as she has heard of other claimants being verbally abused. Although she has considered suicide, her Hindu beliefs have prevented her from acting on them. She is terrified that she will be deported and continues to struggle with a strong sense of worthlessness; thinking that she must be a bad person, 'otherwise, God allow this to happen to me'.

If she could reinvent herself, she would like to be able to develop her skills – perhaps by becoming a teacher of young children – and to be free to express her true self.

Occupational competence

Banita has very little English, no relatives in the UK, and arrived in the UK with just a small suitcase of clothes. She has since received warm clothing from the local

Refugee Action group and has received support to fill out her claim for asylum. The bruises that were on her arms when she arrived in the UK have now healed, but she still has multiple scars from the ill-treatment by her husband. She also had some broken teeth when she arrived, and has been provided with the necessary dental treatment.

Physically, Banita is recovering her strength and has no evident problems. She keeps her room neat and tidy and is proving to be a skilled cook in the house, where the women sometimes prepare meals together and communicate through gestures. Other than mealtimes, however, Banita is spending most of the time in her room and only goes out to buy food or to meet with her solicitor to discuss options for a fresh claim. She is quietly spoken, rarely makes eye contact, and is finding it difficult to get to know people.

Even though Banita explained that she did not own a passport and so the passport she used was not her own, it has become apparent that the Home Office is still calling her by her sister-in-law's name – Yauvani. Subsequently, this is the name that her caseworker and housemates still use. More than this, it means that although Banita brought news clippings with her to prove that her husband was seeking her arrest, they appear to refer to a different person and may be discounted. When the occupational therapist offered to make sure that the documentation was changed, Banita started to make more eye contact and became more open.

Banita's asylum claim was probably refused on the basis that she could have moved to another part of India. At this stage in the claim process, she has been provided with a payment card that can only be used in restricted locations. It is equivalent to 70% of income support and enables her to pay for food and essential toiletries, but she has no way of paying for any more phone calls to her auntie. However, during a recent phone call to her auntie, arranged by a charity worker, it was suggested that her parents may be willing to consider reconciliation.

Key occupational issues

- getting to know people
- expressing true self
- developing skills

Summary statement

Banita is a skilled cook who grew up in India, enjoying art and dancing. Her Hindu faith has kept her going and she dreams of becoming a teacher.

Banita has little English and is currently spending most of her time in her room – struggling to get to know other women in the house and integrating socially in the community. After many years of being confined in an abusive relationship, she wants to be able to express her true self. More than this, she wants the freedom to develop her skills, perhaps by teaching others or working with children.

Initial goals and interventions

1a. Over the next 4 weeks, Banita will plan how to get to know people, with encouragement and suggestions from the occupational therapist (OT)

- Banita to invite her housemates to cook a meal with her
- OT to accompany Banita on walks around the local area
- Banita to talk with caseworker about English lessons
- OT to make contact with the local Hindu community
- Banita to visit local community centre and be introduced to representatives from the Hindu community

2a. Over the next 2 weeks, Banita will identify ways to express her true self, with advocacy from the occupational therapist

- OT and caseworker to arrange for her documentation to be changed to refer to Banita by her own name
- Banita to let her housemates know her true name
- Banita to complete interest checklist with occupational therapist
- OT and Banita to discuss her aspirations, with OT drawing on Cognitive Behavioural Therapy techniques to counter Banita's negative thoughts

3a. Over the next 8 weeks, Banita will explore ways to develop her skills, with direction and structured support from the occupational therapist

- Banita to reflect on opportunities to contribute her skills at the Community Centre
- OT to investigate available opportunities in the local community

Achievements after 3 months

Successive goals were agreed and attained, and Banita's mood was much improved.

- she had begun to forge a close relationship with one of the women she shared a house with
- she was participating in English classes
- she had started teaching Indian Classical Dance to girls at the local community centre
- she and her friend cooked for one another, and sometimes cooked for local charity events
- she is learning how to sew, and is hoping to make clothes for herself
- she even took up swimming, which she had never done before

Box XII.i   An educator's perspective

Learning the skills necessary to construct occupational formulations is extremely valuable for students. It enables you to understand the client's needs in-depth and ensure a truly occupational focus to your work. The more confident you feel about creating a picture of occupational needs the easier it will be for you to translate that understanding into measurable goals and meaningful interventions.

Having a clear formulation also gives you the clarity to be able to articulate your reasoning to the client and others, making the process accessible, and expressing the value of occupation in the client's life.

Table XII.i Components of Banita's occupational identity

Roles/relationships	shunned and threatened by family; moved to live with husband and mother-in-law; worked in new home 'like a slave'; auntie gave her money to fly to the UK; now lives in a house with three other women, none of whom share the same language
Turning points (inc., changes to physical & social environments)	comfortable childhood in India; family wanted an arranged marriage for her; eloped with a man from a different caste; perceived as dishonouring family; mother-in-law started criticising her; did not become pregnant; raped and beaten by husband; took passport belonging to sister-in-law and came to the UK; placed in the NE of England; asylum claim has been refused
Interests	art and dancing. teaching young children
Volition *(inc., appraisal of ability, expectation of success, values, choices, satisfaction & goals)*	fell in love in her teens; sad and ashamed by family's rejection; feared for own life; happily married to begin with; soon felt inadequate and afraid; felt trapped and alone for many years, frightened about travelling to the UK; could not think of what else to do; feels isolated and hopeless; feels self-conscious and afraid when using payment card; considered suicide but prevented by Hindu beliefs; terrified of being deported; feels worthless and bad; would like to develop skills and express true self

Table XII.ii Components of Banita's occupational competence

Routines	sometimes prepares meals with housemates; spends most of time in her room, only going out to buy food or meet with solicitor
Skills	very little English; recovering her strength; communicates with housemates through gestures; quietly-spoken and rarely made eye contact but becoming more open
Performance	keeps room neat and tidy; skilled cook; finding it hard to get to know people
Environmental contexts	no relatives in the UK; small suitcase of clothes; warm clothing from charity; support to claim asylum; dental treatment; solicitor's advice regarding options for fresh claim; Home Office caseworker was still referring to her by her sister-in-law's name; occupational therapist is acting as advocate via Urdu translator; payment card system has been implemented now that asylum claim has been refused; card can be used in limited locations to buy basic necessities, but not phone calls; charity worker arranged recent phone call to auntie; parents may consider reconciliation

Reference

Baron K, Kielhofner G, Iyenger A, Goldhammer V, Wolenski J (2006) *A User's Manual for the Occupational Self Assessment (OSA) Version 2.2*. Chicago: University of Illinois.

XIII Occupational Therapy in an independent vocational service

– an example occupational formulation with measurable goals

Overview

An occupational therapist's role in vocational rehabilitation is based on having an in-depth understanding of the whole person – to get a sense of how the person's life outside of work fits with the work role. At times, there will be occupational issues at home which restrict the person's ability to work, and a well-written formulation will support any decisions that lead to interventions beyond the sphere of work. In this case, Saaid is 'fiercely private', has a home that meets his current needs, and has a degree of social contact and support, but his sedentary lifestyle at home and limited social life may be affecting his health and wellbeing. Through a process of negotiation, he agrees to receive support with two issues that are purely work-related – mobility at work and the office dynamics – and one that includes his life outside work – his work/life balance.

Another person, in similar circumstances, might want to focus more specifically on accessing financial assistance for their mobility needs, developing their assertion skills, and widening their social circle. As the occupational therapist, you need to be skilled in interpreting the people's need and volition, before arriving at three or four issues that encompass all their needs and are worded in a way that will be acceptable to acceptable to them. Agreeing broad issues may confer an advantage as they allow you to offer a range of interventions, some of which will fall by the wayside, while some will prove useful. Ultimately, it is worth remembering that goal attainment is not dependent on the individual interventions being successful, as these are merely the means to an end.

Introduction

Saaid is a 40-year-old man who was diagnosed with Multiple Sclerosis (MS) 5 years ago. He has experienced continence problems, remains at risk of falling, and has periods of low mood. He is working with an independent occupational therapist to resolve vocational issues.

Occupational assessments completed:
- Work Environment Impact Scale (Moore-Corner et al. 1998)
- workplace visit
- non-standardised assessments of transfers, mobility, exercise tolerance, strength and range of movement and dexterity

DOI: 10.4324/9781003046301-113

Notice how:

- the occupational therapist makes use of the Work Environment Impact Scale (Moore-Corner et al. 1998) to gather information about Saaid's job, as well as a variety of non-standardised assessments
- the formulation includes information about Saaid's home-life as well as his work-life
- the summary statement starts with positives about Saaid's identity, followed by a sentence that elaborates on each of the key occupational issues, and Saaid's motivation for addressing each issue is implied by the wording

   o   he *wants* to improve his mobility
   o   he is *unsure* of how to influence the office dynamics
   o   he *would benefit from* a better work/life balance – suggesting that he is not fully convinced of the need to make changes and that further discussion is required. Unsurprisingly, therefore, the first goal associated with this issue is to 're-examine his work/life balance'

- the example goals include a set of initial goals followed by a subsequent set of goals

Occupational identity

Saaid works as an accountant in the payroll department of a large company. It is a job which he knows he does well, but which he often finds tiring. Although he accepts his diagnosis, he feels mortified when he is unable to manage everyday tasks, and describes himself as 'fiercely independent and private'.

He allows everyone at work to call him Sid, and says that he pretends that he is fine. Although he appreciates all the accommodations that have been made at work – including moving his office so that he is closer to suitable toilet facilities where he can change his catheter bag – he 'resents' needing to receive support from his work colleagues. He feels frustrated when they do not appear to appreciate the extent of his problems and irritated by their attempts at humour, which he perceives as bordering on mockery. He often thinks that it would be better to retire on the grounds of ill health.

Saaid is a practising Muslim who took the decision to divorce his wife 6 years ago and prefers not to discuss his family relationships, although he does enjoy Skype-ing his 16-year-old son. Prayers at his local mosque and religious discussions with his Imam have been a source of hope and comfort to him in recent years.

In general, he is fatalistic about what the future holds for him and wants to be 'as normal as possible'.

Occupational competence

Saaid's work has often been praised by his employer, and he is allowed to have flexible working hours so that he can manage his fatigue. He is very methodical, is known for his accuracy, and has no problems with attention or upper body coordination. He is unable to manage getting on and off buses and uses a taxi to get to and from work. He would qualify for financial assistance but is not in receipt of any benefits as yet.

At work, he is able to attend to his continence needs, and has been using a walking stick in the open-plan office. He usually manages to walk around at a slow pace but has experienced several trips and falls while at work, and his manager is concerned about how he would exit the building in an emergency as the office is a long way from the exit. A wheelchair has been provided by the company to be used if needed.

Apparently, when he has lost his balance, his colleagues have laughed and called him a 'clumsy clod' even while they have helped him to his feet. Saaid has laughed with them and is regarded as being 'a good laugh' and someone who joins in the office banter. He has not told them how he feels, but is able to express feelings of irritation and frustration in therapy sessions.

Saaid lives in a bungalow which is suitable for his needs. When at home, he watches the sport on television every night and orders takeaway food online. He has put on two stones (12+ kg) in the past year. He has no contact with his ex-wife, and no-one with whom he confides his feelings, but Skypes his son once every fortnight to see how he is doing. He also attends his mosque once a week, and receives lifts to and from the mosque from members of the congregation.

Key occupational issues

* mobility at work
* office dynamics
* work/life balance

Summary statement

Saaid is a valued accountant in his workplace, where he is considered to be 'a good laugh'. He attends weekly prayers at the mosque, enjoys watching sport on television, and keeps in touch with his son via Skype.

Saaid wants to improve his mobility at work so that he can be as independent as possible and reduce the risk of falling.

He is irritated by his colleagues' jokes about his poor balance and unsure how to influence the office dynamics.

He would benefit from establishing a better work/life balance in which he can socialise and keep as physically active as possible.

Initial goals and interventions

1a. Over the next 4 weeks, Saaid will explore and identify the most suitable options for mobility at work, with information and advice provided by the occupational therapist (OT)

* OT to complete risk assessment of falls and provide relevant advice
* OT to refer to Physiotherapy for assessment and advice on appropriate walking aids
* OT to provide information regarding the possibility of a mobility scooter

- OT to provide information regarding financial support for mobility aids and transport
- OT to discuss advantages and disadvantages of various mobility options

2a. Over the next 2 weeks, Saaid will re-examine and plan possible responses to the office dynamics with encouragement and feedback from the occupational therapist

- OT to encourage reflection on the impact of office dynamics on Saaid's health
- OT to train Saaid in assertive techniques for responding to office dynamics

3a. Over the next 6 weeks, Saaid will re-examine and explore options for improving his work/life balance, in discussion with the occupational therapist

- OT and Saaid to discuss the benefits of increased social and physical activity
- OT to investigate local opportunities for physical exercise and liaise with MS services regarding recommended exercise
- Saaid to investigate social opportunities in the Muslim community and in his workplace

Successive goals and interventions

1b. Within the next 6 weeks, Saaid will independently choose and practise ways to improve mobility at work

- Saaid to trial a mobility scooter

2b. Over the next 8 weeks, Saaid will practise and negotiate ways to respond to the office dynamics, in consultation with his manager

- Saaid to arrange a meeting with his manager to request support for dealing with the office dynamics

3b. Over the next 4 weeks, Saaid will choose and practise ways to improve his work/life balance, with coaching from the occupational therapist

- Saaid to discuss working reduced hours with his manager
- Saaid to try out chosen social and physical activities

Box XIII.i A therapist's perspective

Producing occupational formulations can be such a powerful way of demonstrating to clients your understanding of their occupational identity and occupational competence, whilst teasing out the key occupational issues to help establish meaningful Occupational Therapy goals. It goes far beyond their diagnosis and reason for referral to Occupational Therapy. It can be very satisfying when you receive feedback from clients that you have understood them and how their health conditions are affecting their function in everyday life. More than this, it can be positive and even instrumental in supporting a client's engagement going forward in Occupational Therapy intervention.

Table XIII.i Components of Saaid's occupational identity

Roles/relationships	accountant in payroll department of large company, practising Muslim, divorced 6 years ago; has 16 yr old son
Turning points (inc., changes to physical & social environments)	diagnosed with MS 5 years ago; at risk of falling and has continence problems; accommodations made at work include moving office to be near toilet facilities where he can change his catheter bag; 'resents' needing to receive support from work colleagues
Interests	enjoys skyping his son
Volition *(inc., appraisal of ability, expectation of success, values, choices, satisfaction & goals)*	knows he does job well but finds it tiring; accepts diagnosis but feels mortified when unable to manage tasks; describes self as 'fiercely independent and private'; allows colleagues to call him Sid and pretends he is fine with this; frustrated by lack of appreciation of his problems and irritated by attempts at humour; often thinks of retiring on ill-health grounds; prefers not to discuss family relationships; finds hope and comfort in prayers at local mosque and religious discussions with Imam; fatalistic about the future and wants to be as normal as possible

Table XIII.ii Components of Saaid's occupational competence

Routines	uses a taxi to get to and from work; when at home, watches the sport on television every night; has no contact with ex-wife; attends mosque once a week
Skills	very methodical and accurate; has no problems with attention or upper body coordination; uses walking stick, walking at slow pace, and has had several trips and falls; is regarded as 'a good laugh'; expresses feelings of irritation and frustration in therapy sessions but does not express feelings to anyone else
Performance	unable to manage getting on and off buses; able to attend to his continence needs; orders takeaway food online and has put on two stones (12+ kg) in 1 year
Environmental contexts	lives in bungalow which is suitable for his needs; receives lifts to and from the mosque from members of the congregation; office is open-plan; work is praised by employer; is allowed flexible working hours to manage fatigue; would qualify for financial assistance but hasn't claimed benefits yet; manager is concerned about Saaid exiting the building in an emergency and has arranged for a wheelchair; colleagues laugh and call him clumsy if he trips

Reference

Moore-Corner RA, Kielhofner, G, Olson, L (1998) *A User's Guide to Work Environment Impact Scale (WEIS) Version 2.0.* Chicago: University of Illinois.

XIV Occupational Therapy in an acute physical service

– an example occupational formulation with measurable goals

Overview

If it is difficult to find the time to write a formulation in an acute mental health setting, it is probably even more difficult in acute physical settings, where the emphasis may be on safe discharge and where it is all too easy for occupational therapy to become process-led. Even in this setting, however, if occupational therapists are determined to be person-centred and retain their occupational focus, formulations may enable them to enhance the person's volition and to alert the team to wider issues. In the ideal world, occupational formulations may even allow therapy to be more effective by demonstrating an unmet need for occupational therapists to work with people over a longer time period.

In Courtney's case, the first two issues relate to her skills and task performance, (getting in and out of bed; and washing and dressing her lower body), but the third one acknowledges a much broader issue of participation in a key occupation (re-establishing her role as a mum). The very fact that this last issue is recognised may strengthen Courtney's motivation to work on the first two issues, and it also prompts the occupational therapist to set aside some time to help Courtney to identify her strengths and limitations as a mum; thereby expanding the Occupational Therapy role, which might otherwise have been limited to providing aids and arranging future assistance. It also leads directly into occupation-focused interventions, many of which may be identified by the occupational therapist but carried out by other people after Courtney has been discharged. By taking the time to compose an occupational formulation, the therapist is able to act as an advocate and influence future decisions.

Introduction

Courtney is a 30-year-old woman who was admitted to an acute hospital ward with a severe chest infection and complications due to sleep apnoea. She is being treated for hypertension and has been referred to occupational therapy to address the impact of obesity on her daily activities and quality of life. She weighed 25 stone (160 kg) on admission and is 5 foot 5 inches (165cm) tall. Body Mass Index (BMI) = 58.24

Occupational assessments completed:
* Role Checklist (Scott 2019)
* informal interview and functional assessment, including dressing and transfers

DOI: 10.4324/9781003046301-114

> **Notice how:**
> - the introduction includes a concise overview of Courtney's health conditions, and the occupational formulation is more concise than many other formulations due to the restricted time available
> - the Role Checklist (Scott 2019) has been used to gain a quick understanding of how Courtney's health conditions and her current admission are affecting her life
> - the first two occupational issues focus on specific skills and task performance, and the last one focuses on a broader concern of participation, even though this issue may not be met until after Courtney has been discharged
> - the direct involvement of the occupational therapist is focused primarily on short-term interventions, but the formulation paves the way for future work, including the involvement
>   - o   community Occupational Therapy the Home-Start charity and the possibility of future re-housing

Occupational identity

Courtney is keen to improve her health so that she can look after her three children who are aged 5, 6, and 7. She is a single mum and attributes her over-eating to having had an abusive partner in the past, who criticised the way that she looked and stopped her from leaving the house. He left before her youngest child was born and she is now embarrassed to go out on her own and feels guilty and frustrated because she feels too tired to play with her children.

Her children attend a nearby primary school and walk to school with a group of other children in a 'walking school bus', organised by the Parent-Teacher Association. Courtney does not know how she would manage without this support. When the children are at school she spends time talking to her online friends in an obesity support forum, which she describes as 'a lifeline'. In the past, she has felt trapped and powerless, but she is grateful to the staff at the hospital and is motivated to lose weight in the future. She is excited to be going home to be with her children.

Occupational competence

Courtney's Social Worker describes her as a loving mum, who is gentle and kind. Her children are currently in temporary foster care while she is in the hospital, and will return to live with Courtney with additional support from Social Services. Courtney has no family support and was managing to look after her children by prompting them to complete tasks. Every day after school, she would spend time watching cartoons with them and would order a takeaway meal for them all. When they went to bed she would spend time online.

Courtney lives in an upstairs flat. She experiences joint pain and breathlessness when walking, and before coming to the hospital she had not left the flat for several months. She struggles to get herself in an out of bed, and has difficulty reaching and bending to wash and dress her lower body. She is able to wash and dress her upper body. She needs assistance to manage her hygiene needs and prevent soreness in the folds of her skin. She can mobilise short distances with a frame, and the ward nursing staff have already referred her for Home Care support to assist with domestic tasks. She is also receiving advice from the dietician and physiotherapist, and has already lost 1 stone (2 kg) by following a restricted diet. She is a sociable person who communicates well and has responded positively to professional support.

Key occupational issues

* getting in and out of bed
* washing and dressing lower body
* re-establishing role as mum

Summary statement

Courtney is a loving mum to her three children and is excited to have lost some weight and to be going home. She wants to lose more weight so that she can be more actively involved with her children's care. In order to return home, she will benefit from equipment to help her get in and out of bed. Initially, she will also need assistance to wash and dress her lower body and attend to her hygiene needs. In the long-term, it will be important to support her to re-establish her role as a single mum in her community.

Initial goals and interventions

1. Over the next week, Courtney will practise getting in and out of bed with instruction and supervision from the occupational therapist (OT) and physiotherapist

   * OT to refer to community occupational therapist and forward current occupational formulation
   * OT to provide bed lever and discuss techniques for getting in and out of bed

2. Over the next week, Courtney will practise washing and dressing her lower body with help from the occupational therapy assistant and occupational therapist

   * OT to negotiate assistance required for washing and dressing when Courtney is discharged
   * OT to advise regarding the use and purchase of personal care aids

3. Over the next week, Courtney will identify her strengths and limitations in her role as a mum, and plan activities to strengthen this role, with advice and feedback from the occupational therapist

   * OT and Courtney to spend time examining strengths and limitations during washing and dressing practice
   * OT to liaise with social worker and community OT regarding referral to Home-Start charity
   * OT to discuss possibility of re-housing with the team

Table XIV.i Components of Courtney's occupational identity

Roles/relationships	single mum of three children aged 5, 6 and 7; ex-partner left before youngest was born
Turning points (inc., changes to physical & social environments)	admitted to acute hospital ward with severe chest infection and complications due to sleep apnoea, weighing 25 stone (160 kg); ex-partner criticised the way that she looked and stopped her from leaving the house
Interests	excited to be going home to be with children
Volition *(inc., appraisal of ability, expectation of success, values, choices, satisfaction & goals)*	keen to improve health to look after children; attributes her over-eating to having had an abusive partner; is embarrassed to go out on own, and feels guilty & frustrated as too tired to play with children; does not know how she would manage getting children to and from school without support of the school walking bus; describes online obesity support group as 'a lifeline'; has felt trapped and powerless, but is grateful to hospital staff and motivated to lose weight

Table XIV.ii Components of Courtney's occupational competence

Routines	after school, spent time watching cartoons with children; ordered takeaway meals every day; spent time online once children were in bed; had not left flat for several months
Skills	sociable and communicates well; described by social worker as a loving, kind, gentle mum; can mobilise short distances with a frame; difficulties reaching and bending; experiences joint pain and breathlessness on walking
Performance	was managing to look after her children by prompting them to complete tasks; struggles to get in and out of bed and has difficulty washing and dressing lower body; needs assistance to manage hygiene needs and prevent soreness; has lost 1 stone (2 kg) following a restricted diet
Environmental contexts	continues to have social worker input; children are currently in temporary foster care; no family support; lives in an upstairs flat; ward nursing staff have already referred her for Home Care support to assist with domestic tasks; is receiving advice from the dietician and physiotherapist

Box XIV.i   A manager's perspective

Currently, there is a shift from an illness-based, provider-led system towards one that is patient-led, preventative in focus, that offers care closer to home. Occupational therapists are trained and focused to enable people to live at home and to live well regardless of health or social circumstances. However, in recent years, the pressures of working in health services have created a shift in Occupational Therapy practice from occupational assessments to a focus on the coordination of discharge planning, instead of facilitating early occupational activities. Occupational therapists report that they are doing a considerable amount of discharge coordination and planning with limited opportunities for occupational assessments or interventions.

Occupation formulation provides occupational therapists with a structured framework to guide thier assessment and clinical reasoning, and to articulate the unique assessment of the patient from the perspective of Occupational Therapy. Occupational Therapists need to document their assessment, professional reasoning, and measurable goals in a clear and concise way, so that they are able to demonstrate their unique contribution to the patients' care in a highly pressured environment, and ensure that each patient's occupational identity, competence, and future goals are conveyed to the multi-disciplinary team so that a personalised care plan is developed.

Reference

Scott PJ (2019) *The Role Checklist, Version 3*. Chicago: University of Illinois.

XV Occupational Therapy in a community reablement service

– an example occupational formulation with measurable goals

Overview

This formulation illustrates the complex interaction between physical and mental health, and how Occupational Therapy can offer solutions that will meet the needs of the whole person. Treating the whole person involves paying attention to all their occupational needs, and occupational therapists have long understood that this includes a person's sexual needs. Yet in practice, it seems that many occupational therapists have avoided this topic. Is this because the subject is too sensitive to broach, or is it because the therapists are uncertain of their role and how they might influence a situation?

Imagine a person who is single and who wants to have a loving, intimate relationship with someone. The aim might be for the person to form a loving, intimate relationship – to have a girlfriend or a boyfriend, or to get married, or simply to have sex – but many occupational therapists would struggle to know how to create a measurable goal with a realistic timeframe for the expected outcome. How can anyone tell how long it will take for someone to achieve such goals, and how meaningless would it be to reduce the person's goal to a set of objectives – for example, to focus on their social interaction skills in general, or where they might go to meet someone? These objectives might never lead to the desired relationship and it would be very easy for the therapist to lose sight of the person's dream, and for the person to believe that their ambition was being ignored.

In this formulation, Richard's ill health has affected his marital relationship. The occupational therapist shows how it is possible to negotiate a measurable goal that addresses his concerns, without making any promises about what will happen, and without deviating from the key issue. The dimensions of engagement, as defined by the Model of Human Occupation, (Kielhofner and Forsyth 2008; Pépin 2017) allow the therapist and the person to measure progress in terms of a steady process of change.

Introduction

Richard is a 35-year-old man who always appeared to be very healthy, but developed high blood pressure 1 year ago and was found to have a heart defect. He recently underwent heart surgery to replace a valve and had a stroke after the operation leading to dysphasia (speech problems) and dyspraxia (coordination problems). Once discharged from the hospital, he was referred to the occupational therapist in the Community Reablement service.

DOI: 10.4324/9781003046301-115

Notice how:
- the occupational therapist has conducted assessments related to Richard's symptoms as well as various occupation-focused assessments, but these do not inform the occupational formulation and so have been listed separately
- the ages of Richard's children are stated. This gives the reader a sense of their developmental needs and is in keeping with Child Protection guidelines
- the rehabilitation issues are linked to occupations that are meaningful for Richard rather than focusing on any general matters of skill, such as anyone might experience with similar health problems
- the goals for maintaining a loving relationship as a husband remain focused on the issue rather than deviating to include possible interventions

Occupational assessments completed:
- Occupational Circumstances Assessment Interview and Rating Scale (Forsyth et al. 2005)
- informal functional assessment
- informal interview with wife

+ Depression questionnaire and screening test for hemianopia

Occupational identity

Richard used to be a farmworker and became self-employed 10 years ago, working as a handyman and gardener. He is known locally as 'Mr Fix-It'. He is also a beekeeper and has a smallholding where he keeps goats. He finds it relaxing to milk the nanny goats and has always been very active, enjoying an outdoor life, and playing in local football and cricket teams.

He is married, with one daughter, aged 8, and one son, aged 3, and he misses playing with them and taking them out. He worries about the strain that his ill health has put on his relationship with his wife, and admits to feeling sad that he is no longer the main earner in the household. He would like to show his wife that he still loves her, and keeps cheerful for his family's sake.

He used to enjoy reading – mainly about beekeeping, goat husbandry, plumbing, and electrics – and currently says he has no interest in reading or in watching television. He is grateful for the company of his friends in the village and feels frustrated when he cannot find the right words in a conversation. He describes his friends as 'the salt of the earth', who would do anything for him, and in the future, he hopes to take up golf with them.

Occupational competence

Richard's wife and his friends take him to see his goats every day, and his friends have set up a rota to tend the goats. Richard has proved able to milk the goats and supervise any work that needs to be done, but is unable to participate in any strenuous exercise while his chest wall heals. He has difficulty with tasks that require fine motor control but has already made good progress and is now able to dress himself and manage all his personal activities of daily living.

Richard spends much of the day watching over his son while he plays, and his children seem to have adapted to him being ill and appear to enjoy having him at home. His wife's cake-making business is doing well, and so she and Richard are able to manage financially for the time being. His wife feels that she has to stay strong for the family and she is doing all she can to find out about Richard's health needs. She acknowledges that she sometimes feels more like Richard's carer and would like to feel more like his wife. They have refrained from having an intimate relationship since Richard's diagnosis last year.

Richard remains very emotional at times, which is common after a stroke. He also muddles his words at times but is very expressive with his hands and is able to communicate his thoughts and feelings, and to joke with his friends. Physically, he is out of condition, having spent a year not working, and he is gradually regaining strength.

Key occupational issues

- contributing to the home and family – now and the future
- regaining physical fitness to play golf
- maintaining a loving relationship as a husband

Summary statement

Richard is known locally as 'Mr Fix-It'. He is a self-employed handyman and gardener, who also keeps goats and bees.

While he is recovering from heart surgery and a stroke, it is important for him to be able to contribute to his home and family by identifying the jobs that he can still do and retaining his work role. He has always been active and played sports (including football and cricket), and hopes to be able to play golf with his friends. More than anything, he would like to maintain a loving relationship with his wife, who has done so much to support him.

Initial goals and interventions

1a. Within 2 weeks, I will identify how I can make contributions to my home and family, with suggestions from the occupational therapist (OT)

- OT to check that Richard understands which activities he needs to avoid
- OT and Richard to create a list of gentle activities to pursue with son and daughter, practising fine coordination where possible
- Richard to participate in meal preparation activities graded by the OT
- OT to instruct Richard in exercises using therapeutic putty, including making play shapes for his son

2a. Over the next 6 weeks, I will practise skills necessary for playing golf, with instruction from the occupational therapist

- OT to plan graded walking programme and discuss activities that Richard can practise while tending his goats and bees

3a. Over the next 2 weeks, I will plan ways to be a loving husband with reassurance and advice from my occupational therapist

- OT to provide Richard with information about sexual activity after heart surgery and provide counselling for Richard and his wife
- OT to discuss ideas with Richard for expressing romantic love

Successive goals and interventions *(in order, as negotiated)*

1b. Over the next 4 weeks, I will plan and practise contributions to my home and family with encouragement from my occupational therapist

- Richard to walk his daughter to school each day
- Richard to commence gentle gardening and maintenance activities and structured bilateral exercises

3b. Over the next 10 weeks, I will maintain a loving relationship as a husband with reassurance from my occupational therapist

- OT to review Richard's progress and liaise with speech and language therapist regarding Richard's communication

1c. Over the next 6 weeks, I will explore further ways to contribute to the home and family, with coaching from my occupational therapist
- Richard is investigating making cheese using goats milk

2b. Over the next 6 weeks, I will re-examine and practise further skills for playing golf, in a graded programme supervised by my occupational therapist

- Richard to continue bilateral exercises
- Richard to accompany his friends to a 9-hole golf course. Friends to carry equipment and Richard to practise putting

Box XV.i   A manager's perspective

Clinical notes are a snapshot in time of the person. Occupational formulations reflect a fuller picture of the person: their identity (past and present), their valued occupations, and chosen goals. This is in contrast to many clinical notes by multidisciplinary team members regarding diagnosis, current and past symptoms. They motivate both service users and staff members to hold onto a wider vision, despite the challenges that exist for the person and the barriers in the environment. These barriers may include a risk assessment focus and a corresponding absence of positive risk-taking to enhance quality of life.

Over time, I have found that occupational formulation and measurable goals have changed the focus of interventions. The clear goals have enhanced the occupational therapists' ability to work on person-centred goals and not be distracted from their intention. This has enhanced the quality of the Occupational Therapy service.

Table XV.i   Components of Richard's occupational identity

Roles/relationships	worked as farmworker and now self-employed handyman and gardener; known as 'Mr Fix it'; married, with one daughter, aged 8, and one son, aged 3; enjoys company of village friends
Turning points (inc., changes to physical & social environments)	became self-employed 10 years ago; heart defect discovered last year leading to heart surgery followed by stroke
Interests	keeping bees and goats on a smallholding; used to enjoy reading – mainly about beekeeping and goat husbandry, plumbing and electrics; currently has no interest in reading or in watching television; used to play in local football and cricket teams
Volition *(inc., appraisal of ability, expectation of success, values, choices, satisfaction & goals)*	valued being active and outdoor life, and found milking nanny goats was relaxing; misses playing with children and taking them out; worries about the strain his ill health puts on his relationship with his wife; feeling sad that no longer the main earner; would like to show his love to wife and keep cheerful for his family's sake; feels frustrated when he cannot find words; values friends who would do anything for him; hopes to take up golf with them

Table XV.ii   Components of Richard's occupational competence

Routines	sees goats every day; spends rest of the day watching over his son; has refrained from intimate relations with wife since diagnosis
Skills	difficulty with tasks requiring fine motor control; very emotional at times and muddles his words but expressive with hands and able to communicate thoughts and feelings and joke with friends; out of condition physically but is gradually regaining strength
Performance	has spent a year not able to work; now able to milk the goats and supervise work on smallholding; also able to dress self and manage personal activities of daily living; unable to do any strenuous exercise while his chest wall heals
Environmental contexts	wife and friends take him to the smallholding and friends have a rota to tend the goats; children have adapted to him being ill and enjoy having him at home; wife's cake-making business is doing well, and they are managing financially; wife feels she has to stay strong and is researching his health needs; she sometimes feels more like a carer than a wife

References

Forsyth K, Deshpande S, Kielhofner G, Henrikson C, Haglund L, Olson L, Skinner S, Kulkarni S (2005) *The Occupational Circumstances Assessment Interview and Rating Scale (OCAIRS) Version 4.0*. Chicago: University of Illinois.

Kielhofner G, Forsyth K (2008) Occupational engagement: how clients achieve change. In: Kielhofnered G, ed. *Model of Human Occupation: Theory and Application*. 4th ed. Baltimore: Lippincott, Williams & Wilkins.101–09.

Pépin G, (2017) Occupational engagement: how clients achieve change. In: Taylor RR, ed. *Kielhofner's Model of Human Occupation*. 5th ed. Philadelphia: Wolters Kluwer. 187–94.

XVI Occupational Therapy in an adult social care service

– an example occupational formulation with measurable goals

Overview

Here is an interesting formulation, one which manages to affirm the person's identity, even though the remit of the occupational therapist is limited to environmental adaptations. The remit might have been wider if Frances' rehabilitation needs were not already being attended to and if the budgets for Social Services were more extensive, but the occupational therapist still has a very important role in helping Frances to meet her goals. Sharing this formulation provides an opportunity to:

- build trust, by signalling the therapist's intention to treat Frances as an individual
- remind everyone who becomes involved in Frances' care that her identity is more than a wheelchair-user with a C6 spinal lesion
- prompt others to have meaningful conversations with Frances in the future
- explain how the occupational therapist's role links to Frances' rehabilitation needs in a concise and readily understandable format

The formulation reads more like a formal contract than a treatment plan, because all the goals are for the occupational therapist to complete. This is an option that might be used when people lack the capacity to understand an abstract goal, as it still allows clinicians to measure whether or not therapy is making a difference. Even though this is not the case in this scenario, the goals have the advantage of showing that the occupational therapist intends to alleviate Frances' stress by taking the bulk of the responsibility for the actions. The importance of consulting with Frances and her wife, Danielle, is not forgotten, and they will be consulted at every stage to make sure that their specific requirements are met whenever possible.

Introduction

Frances is a 42-year-old woman who sustained a C6 spinal cord injury 8 months ago when she mistakenly dived into the shallow end of a swimming pool. She was admitted to a Spinal Cord Injury Centre 7 months ago, following orthopaedic surgery at an acute hospital; and 4 weeks ago, she was transferred to a residential unit because her home was no longer suitable for her needs. The Adult Social Care Occupational Therapy service is now involved in assessing her needs at home, including the need for home modifications, with the expectation that major adaptations may be required.

DOI: 10.4324/9781003046301-116

Notice how:

- it has been stipulated that the Key Issues, which are all environmental, are those that will be addressed by the Adult Social Care service, leaving the way open for further issues to be addressed by other services
- all the goals are for the occupational therapist to complete
- each goal is linked with an action that involves respecting Frances' choices, discussing options with Frances, and consulting with Frances and her wife
- listing all the interventions in relation to each goal demonstrates the impressive extent of the occupational therapists role
- when analysing the components of Frances' Occupational Identity, the narrative emphasises a multitude of turning points that have affected her life in the last year alone; and when analysing the components of her Occupational Competence, the therapist highlights the many environmental factors that will influence the treatment plan

Occupational assessments completed:

- Occupational Circumstances Assessment Interview and Ratings Scale (OCAIRS) – with recommended questions for Physical Settings (Forsyth et al. 2005)
- home assessment

Occupational identity

Until Frances' accident, she worked in her dream job as a flight attendant for a major airline. She met her wife, Danielle, at work when she was 30 and says that they have made 'the perfect team'. Danielle has decided to take early retirement to care for Frances, and Frances worries about being a burden but also feels that they can manage anything together. Danielle has now arranged the sale of their inner-city flat and, having sought advice, she has bought a dormer bungalow that is suitable for adaptation, and Frances is excited to move into their new home.

The last 2 years have not been easy for the couple, as both Frances' mum and step-dad died following periods of ill-health, and it was hard to balance work and caring responsibilities, especially since Frances has no siblings who could have helped her. Travelling to see her parents when they were ill was very time-consuming, as Frances does not drive, and , following their death she and Danielle had been looking forward to having more time together. Inheritance money allowed them to buy their first house instead of renting, and they moved in just a few months before Frances was paralysed.

Understandably, Frances feels that living in the residential unit is depressing but, on the whole, she has come to terms with her accident. She also takes full responsibility for it happening as she was 'tipsy' at the time. She was always interested in travel, fashion, and cooking and cannot wait to personalise her new home with the small amount of savings left over from the latest house purchase. She has no wish to learn to drive an adapted car, but otherwise wants to be as independent as possible, and is gaining confidence in using a wheelchair and in managing most activities of daily living. It is also important to Frances to be 'as chic as possible', and she is determined to live life to the fullest.

Occupational competence

Frances has made good progress since her accident. Her legs and torso are paralysed and she has difficulty straightening her elbows, but she can bend her elbows and oppose her fingers and thumbs. She lacks wrist stability and strength in her hands and has been provided with orthoses that allow her to feed herself, wash her face, brush her teeth, write, and type. She can also propel a manual wheelchair for short distances indoors, and operate a power-assisted wheelchair. In addition, she can perform level transfers using a transfer board and turn in bed with the use of side rails. Her airline colleagues have already started fundraising on social media to raise money for any specialist equipment that Frances may need.

The residential unit is 40 miles from Frances's new home – a dormer bungalow with space to convert a downstairs reception room into a bedroom. The bathroom upstairs and the downstairs toilet is not accessible using a wheelchair, but it should be possible to convert a utility room into a shower room, adjoining the new bedroom. Other than this, there is sufficient living space on the ground floor, which is level and mostly open-plan. Access to the front-door is currently via three steps and there may be insufficient space for a ramp, so further assessment is needed. Once through the house, however, a patio area can be accessed via bi-fold doors.

With regard to financial matters, Frances did not have relevant insurance coverage and is not pursuing compensation. In the meantime, Danielle has been advised by the Rehabilitation team to apply for a Carer's Allowance. She manages to visit Frances almost every day to assist with daily care – including catheterisation and bowel care, as well as pressure management.

Frances has already researched and acquired fashionable clothing to wear, and has proven able to cook and perform light housework. While she makes the transition to her new home, she will continue to benefit from outreach rehabilitation by the Spinal Injuries Unit to optimise her upper limb function. In the future, she would benefit from having fixtures and fittings adapted to wheelchair height, and advice regarding how to access potential funding for any further equipment needs.

Key occupational issues to be addressed by social services

- adapting downstairs accommodation
- enabling wheelchair access to the front door
- advising about funding for future needs

Summary statement

Frances is interested in travel, fashion, and cooking, and is determined to live life to the fullest in her new home with her wife. She has already made good progress, using a wheelchair and managing everyday tasks, and continues to receive support from the Rehabilitation Outreach team.

Frances' downstairs accommodation requires adapting to create a downstairs bedroom with accessible shower and toilet, and her front door is currently accessed via three steps and must be transformed to become wheelchair accessible. Her airline colleagues are fundraising via social media, but she will also benefit from advice regarding funding for future equipment needs.

Initial goals and interventions

1a. Over the next 4 weeks, the Social Services occupational therapist will plan how to adapt Frances' downstairs accommodation
   The occupational therapist will

- create a design brief based on the specifications and dimensions of the property

   o   for a downstairs bedroom and bathroom
   o   for wheelchair accessible fixtures and fittings
      ■   to prioritise enabling Frances to cook independently, including lowered surfaces and adjustable height for the sink
- consult Frances' wishes at all stages of the adaptation and respect her choices regarding layout and style
- apply for a Disabled Facilities grant and investigate options for topping up grant funding if needed
- liaise with all relevant parties including the surveyor and architect as required
- make recommendations for modifications that take a strengths-based approach, and adhere to current policy guidelines regarding cost-effectiveness

2a. Over the next 2 weeks, the Social Services occupational therapist will identify the most suitable way to provide wheelchair access to Frances' front door
   The occupational therapist will

- check exact measurements for a potential ramp, and if space allows arranging for a temporary ramp whilst major adaptations are progressed
- if a ramp is not possible due to space constraints, investigate the provision of a step lift
- discuss potential options with Frances and Danielle

3a. Over the next 8 weeks, the Social Services occupational therapist and Frances will explore options for funding future needs
   The occupational therapist will

- liaise with Social Work colleagues
- consult with Frances and her wife, and liaise with the rehabilitation occupational therapists to anticipate unmet needs

   o   work with rehabilitation therapist to implement a fatigue management plan
   o   consider hoisting options if transfers become too exhausting

- o   investigate funding for cars that accommodate a wheelchair, with Danielle as the driver

- share information about benefits advice, Personal Care budgets and Direct Payments

  - o   if agreed with Frances and Danielle, liaise with Social Workers to secure a Personal Care budget for additional support

- provide information regarding assistive technology, e.g., specialist alarm/alert systems that may support independence, as well as the technology available on the open market
- liaise with the outreach rehabilitation team and start the conversation regarding future occupations and potential for employment

---

Box XVI.i   A therapist's perspective

Developing skills in occupational formulation and measurable goal setting, within the MOHO framework, has enabled me to enhance my practice. It has allowed me to focus on a person's Occupational Therapy needs when faced with many other competing demands. I now work in an occupationally focused way first and foremost, and thinking about the other ways that I could support or signpost the person is secondary to this.

In my experience, occupational formulation is an open and honest way of working in collaboration with the service user.

- it helps set a clear way forward in the treatment pathway, where both the therapist and service user sign up to developing a plan towards discharge, and both have a copy of the documentation
- it has even helped identify when someone is not ready to make changes at that point in time, and whether they might benefit from being referred back to the service in the future

In addition, having formal reports that state a person's goal attainment provides non-Occupational Therapy managers with powerful evidence that Occupational Therapy interventions have been completed successfully. And in the long run, I believe that occupational formulation clarifies the Occupational Therapist's scope of practice in the MDT in relation to other professionals, and how we can contribute towards care in a unique way.

Table XVI.i Components of Frances's occupational identity

Roles/relationships	worked as flight attendant for major airline; wife to Danielle; only child to mum and step-dad; carer for parents; not a driver
Turning points (inc., changes to physical & social environments)	parents died after period of ill-health; inheritance monies allowed purchase of inner-city flat; diving accident led to C6 spinal injury and admission to rehabilitation unit; wife took early retirement;

	property was unsuitable for a wheelchair user; transferred from rehabilitation unit to residential home; dormer bungalow purchased
Interests	travel, fashion and cooking
Volition *(inc., appraisal of ability, expectation of success, values, choices, satisfaction & goals)*	flight attendant role was dream job; wife and herself make 'the perfect team'; worries about being a burden but feels they can manage anything together; last 2 years have not been easy; was looking forward to having time with wife; living in residential unit is depressing; cannot wait to personalise new home; no wish to learn to drive an adapted car; wants to be as independent and as 'chic' as possible; is gaining confidence in wheelchair use and managing ADLs; determined to live life to the full

Table XVI.ii Components of Frances's occupational competence

Routines	wife visits most days and assists with daily care, including catheterisation, bowel care & pressure management
Skills	legs and torso are paralysed; difficulty straightening elbows, but can bend them; can oppose fingers & thumbs; lacks wrist stability & hand strength;
Performance	has made good progress; able to feed self, wash face, brush teeth, write and type; able to propel wheelchair for short distances indoors; performs level transfers; able to turn in bed; can cook and do light housework
Environmental contexts	manual and power-assisted wheelchairs; orthoses to support wrist stability and hand strength; transfer board; side rails for bed; colleagues have started fundraising for specialist equipment e.g., car to accommodate wheelchair; residential unit is 40 miles from new home; dormer bungalow has space to convert downstairs room into bedroom, and utility room into shower room; ground floor has sufficient space for wheelchair, front door access has three steps; rear patio can be accessed by bi-fold doors; carer's allowance awaited; outreach rehabilitation to continue; would benefit from adapted fixtures & fittings and funding advice

Reference

Forsyth K, Deshpande S, Kielhofner G, Henrikson C, Haglund L, Olson L, Skinner S, Kulkarni S (2005) *The Occupational Circumstances Assessment Interview and Rating Scale (OCAIRS) Version 4.0.* Chicago: University of Illinois.

XVII Occupational Therapy in an intermediate care service

– an example occupational formulation with measurable goals

Overview

The older a person is, the formulation will need to represent a wealth of information relating to past roles, relationships, and interests. In this way, it attempts to convey the richness of the person's life story and all the facets that have contributed to the person's occupational identity. These details will enable staff members to initiate meaningful conversations with the person and forge person-centred relationships.

This formulation differs from all the other ones in the book – which were co-created to represent reality, but are based on fictional particulars – in that it describes the experiences of a real person who gave his permission for the occupational formulation to be included as it is. When you read the Introduction and see that Mr J's admission was triggered by a fall from his mobility scooter, you might assume that he would not want to drive his scooter again. How wrong you would be! The formulation makes it clear that Mr J is a confident, sociable person who enjoys being outdoors, and who wants to return to his previous level of independence which includes going out on a scooter.

By negotiating a key issue focusing on Mr J's use of his mobility scooter, his treatment plan became much more motivating than it would have been if it had focused on skills such as strength and balance, or on the intervention of falls management. The fact that Mr J agreed that the occupational therapist could submit the formulation for inclusion in the book, is a testament to the skills of the occupational therapist in capturing his viewpoint and articulating his needs.

Introduction

Mr J is an 85-year-old man with multiple conditions; pulmonary fibrosis, arthritis, ischaemic heart disease, rheumatic fever, and multiple drug allergies. Following a fall from his mobility scooter 5 weeks ago, he was initially managed at home and then admitted to hospital 3 weeks ago due to worsening pain.

He was treated in the hospital for a right pubic rami fracture, urine retention, and a chest infection, and then referred to Social Care for ongoing rehabilitation and admitted to an Intermediate Care Unit for assessment of his ability to return home.

DOI: 10.4324/9781003046301-117

Assessments completed:
* informal interview and functional assessment

+ Mini-Mental State Examination (MMSE) (Folstein et al. 1975)

Notice how:
* the assessments do not include a formal occupational assessment. Standardised assessments, although useful, are not essential
* although the previous five formulations list three key occupational issues each, this formulation merits four key issues, due to the complexity of the case and the breadth of the occupational therapist's role
* the key issues start with the one that seems to be the most important to Mr J – being able to go out on his mobility scooter again

    o   this goal does not guarantee that he will return to using his scooter, but helps him to move towards his preferred outcome
    o   were he to re-evaluate the goal and decide that it was not realistic, then subsequent goals could be broadened to 'going out' in general

* even though the actions associated with the third issue, adapting the home environment, rely on the interventions of the occupational therapist, the goal itself is still worded to involve Mr J in its completion, as the options are to be *negotiated* with him

---

Occupational identity

Mr J was brought up and stayed in the local area, and was in the Royal Air Force before working in the Police Force until he had Rheumatic fever. He then became a Health and Safety Advisor in a factory, having studied management at university. The job could often be stressful and he retired some 20 years ago. Since then, he has built up an array of hobbies. He is an avid reader and, among other things he enjoys painting, researching local history, model-making, collecting model vehicles, writing, and completing puzzles. He also enjoyed being outdoors on his mobility scooter.

He lives on his own, having been widowed after 61 years of marriage, and although he feels down at times he has 'just got on with things' since then. He used to go out socialising with his wife and friends but says people tend to come to see him now. He is in contact with his three grown children, a brother, a sister-in-law, and various grandchildren, whom he enjoys seeing.

Mr J prefers to spend his time alone in his room on the Unit as he feels unable to relate to some of the other more cognitively impaired patients here. He demonstrates good insight into his current abilities and recognises that he will need some support at home – at least initially – as he is keen not to fall again. He hopes to return to his previous level of independence and would like to get back to using his mobility scooter again. He feels optimistic that he will be able to cook for himself and tidy up around the house, as well as being able to shower and take his medication.

Occupational competence

Mr J lived on his own prior to his fall and was independent with personal care and showering. He is still able to participate in some of his hobbies while in intermediate care, and his house is full of displays of his work and models that he was completing.

Mr J was previously out on his scooter or with family three to four times a week, and has always maintained contact with his brother and his children. His family visits him regularly in the Intermediate Care Unit and Mr J is observed to have good relationships with them. Prior to his fall they helped with shopping, cleaning, and laundry and will continue to help out in the future.

Mr J is making steady progress with his mobility and currently needs the assistance of one person to complete personal care tasks as he has difficulty reaching down to wash and dress himself. With the assistance of two people to transfer from sitting to standing, he can walk for 10 metres with a Zimmer frame and take himself to the toilet in his room.

Mr J has no memory problems and is able to self-medicate on the Unit. He scored 29/30 on an MMSE here. He has participated in various group tasks and has managed independently to make a hot drink, but would benefit from further practice prior to discharge. He is mainly limited by the pain in his back and left side following his fracture.

Assessment has indicated that Mr J will require some support and modification of his home environment to live at home, as there is a large step into his house, he has a very low armchair and several items of furniture will need moving so that he can use his Zimmer frame.

Key occupational issues

- returning to going out on his mobility scooter
- returning to his previous interests and hobbies
- adapting home environment
- managing personal care

Summary statement

Mr J is a retired Health and Safety Advisor, and prior to his fall and subsequent fracture, he enjoyed visits from his family, being outdoors on his mobility scooter, reading, model-making, painting, and completing puzzles.

He has worked hard to regain his mobility but would currently have difficulty transferring onto his scooter. He is determined to return to his previous levels of independence once home and take up all his hobbies again. Mr J's home will require some modification and he will need some practical support at least initially at discharge to manage his personal care.

Initial goals and interventions

1a. Over the next 4 weeks, Mr J will practise transfers with a view to returning to use his mobility scooter, initially with advice and assistance of two staff members, and reviewed by the Occupational Therapist (OT)

- OT to oversee ongoing therapy to improve Mr J's mobility and assess progress with walking

- OT to review transfers on/off bed and chair

2a. Over the next 4 weeks, Mr J will identify and sustain some of his usual hobbies with encouragement from the Occupational Therapist and support from family to access resources

- Mr J to ask family to bring books and puzzles into the unit

3a. Within the next 4 weeks, Mr J will negotiate options for home adaptations with advice and necessary referrals made by the Occupational Therapist

- OT to recommend referral to a service that will remove the existing step into the house and replace with two smaller steps
- OT to recommend that family remove or relocate items of furniture to improve access throughout the house
- OT to refer Mr J for 12-inch grab rail by his bed if required

4a. Over the first 4 weeks of admission, Mr J will practise personal care with the assistance of one staff member, monitored by the Occupational Therapist

- OT to refer for toilet frame as needed
- OT to suggest use of a commode or urine bottle during the day-time, and using stairlift only with supervision in the morning and evening
- OT to refer to Community Therapy to assess accessing the shower once Mr J is at home

Possible future goals

1b. Over the next 4 weeks, Mr J will continue to re-examine his ability to use his mobility scooter, with feedback from the Community Occupational Therapist
2b. Within 4 weeks, Mr J will sustain previous meaningful interests at home with guidance from Community Occupational Therapist
3b. Over the next 4 weeks, Mr J will identify any further home adaptations required, with advice from the Community Occupational Therapist
4b. Over the next 4 weeks of admission, Mr J will practise personal care tasks at home with supervision and prompts from one person
1c. Over the next 4 weeks, Mr J will plan and practise a graded return to using his mobility scooter, with advice from the Community Occupational Therapist

Box XVII.i   Therapists' perspectives

Occupational formulation has helped us structure discussion of people we support in a more objective and occupation-centred manner.

The discussion of the occupational formulation with the person also helps us validate the information we have gathered and cement our person-centred practice.

Occupational formulation has helped us to measure the person's progress in supervision, however small, more accurately.

Table XVII.i Components of Mr J's occupational identity

Roles/relationships	was in the RAF and Police Force before becoming a Health and Safety Advisor in a factory; widowed, having been married for 61 years; has three grown children, grandchildren, and a brother and sister-in-law; used to socialise with wife and friends, and people come to see him now
Turning points (inc., changes to physical & social environments)	left the Police Force after having Rheumatic Fever and studied Management at University; retired 20 years ago; living on own after wife died; fell off mobility scooter and fractured pelvis; initially managed at home; admitted due to worsening pain
Interests	reading, painting, researching local history, model-making, collecting model vehicles, writing and completing puzzles
Volition *(inc., appraisal of ability, expectation of success, values, choices, satisfaction & goals)*	enjoyed being outdoors on mobility scooter; feels down at times but has 'just got on with things'; enjoys seeing family; prefers to spend time alone on the Unit as feels unable to relate to some of the other patients; good insight and recognises he will need some support at home; keen not to fall again; hopes to return to previous level of independence using his mobility scooter; feels optimistic about ability to cook, tidy shower and take medication

Table XVII.ii Components of Mr J's occupational competence

Routines	used to go out on scooter or with family 3-4 times a week; family are visiting regularly; is now participating in various group tasks and practising independent living tasks
Skills	has good relationships with family; is making steady progress with mobility; has difficulty reaching down to wash and dress himself; can walk for 10 metres with a Zimmer frame; has no memory problems (scoring 29/30 on an MMSE)
Performance	currently needs assistance of one person to complete personal care tasks; requires assistance of two people to transfer from sitting to standing so that he can go to the toilet; is able to self-medicate on the unit; has managed independently to make a hot drink; mainly limited by pain in back and left side following fracture
Environmental contexts	family helped with shopping, cleaning and laundry and will continue to help in future; he will require some support and modification of home environment due to steps into his house, very low armchair, and items of furniture need moving to allow for Zimmer frame

Reference

Folstein MF, Folstein SE, McHugh PR (1975) 'Mini-mental status'. A practical method for grading the cognitive state of patients for the clinician. *Journal of Psychiatric Research*, *12(3)*, 189–98.

XVIII Occupational Therapy in a dementia assessment service

– an example occupational formulation with measurable goals

Overview

When occupational therapists are tasked with discharge-planning, as is often the case, then it is essential to present all the relevant information in a coherent way, allowing everyone involved to make an informed decision. Occupational formulations enable this brief to be met by synthesising all the relevant details into a comprehensive narrative; spanning past and present circumstances, and contrasting the person's subjective viewpoint with an objective account of what is happening.

In this formulation, the goals are set, not for Bob or for the individual occupational therapist, but for the occupational therapy and the multi-disciplinary team. For this reason, it is essential that the whole team gains an understanding of Bob's needs, and that plans are comprehensible to Bob's family. The occupational formulation provides an excellent vehicle for gathering and sharing knowledge by giving a vivid account of Bob's occupational life and his occupational performance. It helps everyone to understand that many of the behaviours that they might find challenging are rooted in Bob's past routines, and in his continuing need to keep active and be involved in productive tasks.

Although the occupational therapist takes responsibility for composing the formulation and will contribute his or her own observations, the content of the formulation can be drawn from the findings of everyone involved. The therapist may even facilitate a formulation meeting to gather information about clients – to corroborate information about their roles, relationships, life turning points, interests and goals, and to confirm observations about their skills, routines, abilities, and the environmental context.

Introduction

Bob is an 80-year-old gentleman who was diagnosed with Alzheimer's disease 4 years ago. He has difficulty hearing and presents with some expressive dysphasia. Since being admitted to an assessment unit, he has been treated for a chest infection, an ear infection, and cellulitis. He was also automatically referred to occupational therapy for an assessment of his occupational needs to inform discharge planning.

Occupational assessments completed:
- Model of Human Occupation Exploratory Level Outcome Ratings (MOHO-ExpLOR) (Cooper et al. 2018)
- informal interview with wife, based on the Occupational Performance History Interview (OPHI) (Kielhofner et al. 2004)

DOI: 10.4324/9781003046301-118

Notice how:

- knowledge of Bob's identity relies on information provided by his family, with detailed evidence of his roles and routines gathered by using aspects of the Occupational Performance History Interview
- the Occupational Therapy support staff have noticed how Bob responds to their interactions, and their observations have been included in the Competence section
- whereas some treatment plans might be worded as problems – e.g., 'communication is inconsistent', 'Bob's dignity is compromised', 'Bob's actions can lead to damage and obstruction', and 'a long-term care setting has not been identified' – the key occupational issues are all phrased positively
- the interventions are to be completed in collaboration with either the nursing team, the OT support staff, the physiotherapist or the whole multi-disciplinary team (MDT)

Occupational identity

Bob was brought up on a farm, and for many years he worked as a shepherd and farm manager. Until recently, he lived with his wife Alwynne on a smallholding. They are very private, stoic, and independent people who prefer to 'get by' without help, and have kept many of their difficulties to themselves.

Bob was described by his family as a quiet, reserved, placid gentleman, who enjoyed the outdoor life, walking, and reading non-fiction. He would attend village social events with his wife but was also happy in his own company, and liked to keep himself busy with jobs around the smallholding.

Although they no longer keep livestock, Bob used to take great care to ensure the welfare of his animals and had a close bond with his sheepdog. He was used to being his own boss and ensuring that farmhands did their work satisfactorily. He coped with the long hours and unpredictable routines at lambing time, and he would wash his hands in streams and troughs when out in the fields. When assisting with morning milking, he would dress in clean overalls which would require changing afterwards.

When first admitted, he was unsettled and angry towards staff and frustrated by any in-terventions. His preferences are now becoming apparent: he is inclined to participate in work-like activities, and prefers to be in quiet places, often choosing to sit outside in the courtyard.

Occupational competence

Bob's admission was triggered by Alwynne being admitted to hospital for a short period following a fall. Bob was placed in emergency care in a nearby residential home and it quickly became apparent that his dementia was much more advanced than had previously been thought, and the home was unable to meet Bob's needs. Bob became aggressive at times and withdrawn at others, sitting with his eyes closed.

Bob has a large and supportive family, but the assessment unit is a long way from his home and his family cannot visit as often as they would like. Moreover, he appears not to recognise his wife and children, and will often get up and walk away when they visit. Mostly, he keeps himself to himself and does not relate to others spontaneously, often taking his meals to eat on his own. However, he is responsive to interaction that is initiated by the occupational therapy support staff – looking at farming magazines and a photo of his favourite sheepdog, Bess, and he shows humour at times.

Bob is a physically strong man of imposing stature and is independently mobile despite having an unsteady gait due to swollen feet. In the days following admission he was wakeful and agitated at night, but has now settled into a routine of going to bed at midnight, rising at 5 AM and napping occasionally during the day. He eats well and can be prompted to participate in self-care activities, but there are also times when he undresses and urinates in public areas, resisting staff intervention when they attempt to maintain his dignity, and before becoming physically and verbally aggressive.

The ward environment is specifically designed for people with dementia, and its design facilitates Bob to walk around the unit. He is always doing something. He becomes focused on the tasks in hand and has inadvertently damaged objects or caused obstructions. He has been observed taking the cushion pads out of their covers and trying to put the covers back on, moving walking frames, and attempting to mend objects around the ward. These are not goal-directed but demonstrate his ability to engage in meaningful activity.

Key occupational issues

- establishing clear communication
- maintaining Bob's dignity
- involving Bob in goal-directed, work-like activities
- identifying a long-term care setting

Summary statement

Bob has spent all his life on farms, and was a quiet, reserved gentleman who enjoyed the outdoor life, walking, and reading non-fiction.

Bob has difficulty hearing others and expressing himself, and sometimes undresses and urinates in public areas. Care needs to be taken to establish clear communication with him and maintain his dignity. He likes to keep busy doing work-like activities and, without direction, he can damage objects or cause obstructions. Any future care setting will need to facilitate goal-directed activities, as well as allowing his family to visit more easily than they can at present.

Initial goals and interventions

1a. Over the next week, the occupational therapy team will identify ways to establish clear communication with Bob, in collaboration with the nursing team

- all staff to be on Bob's right-hand side when talking to him and to supplement verbal communication with clear gestures
- nursing staff to refer Bob to audiology
- picture of Bob's farmhouse to be placed on the door to Bob's room

2a. Over the next 2 weeks, the occupational therapy team will plan how to maintain Bob's dignity, in collaboration with the nursing team

- occupational therapist to ask Bob's family to bring in a pair of clean overalls that Bob can take on and off over his clothes
- nursing staff to put a plan in place for asking Bob if he needs the toilet at key points throughout the day, and showing him where the toilet is

3a. Over the next 3 weeks, the occupational therapy (OT) team will explore options for engaging Bob in goal-directed, work-like activities

- OT support staff to spend 5–10 minutes with Bob every day, looking at farming magazines and photos of his favourite sheepdog, Bess
- OT support staff to invite Bob to take part in gardening activities including sweeping and general maintenance activities in the courtyard
- occupational therapist and physiotherapist to invite Bob to take part in physical exercise groups
- occupational therapist to teach Bob's family how to create a Life History book
- occupational therapist to work with Bob's family to produce a 'rummage box' with memorabilia and small implements that can be handled safely
- Bob to be introduced to the Pets-as-Therapy volunteer
- if possible, occupational therapist to check how Bob responds to being offered a toy sheepdog to hold

4a. Within 3 weeks, the occupational therapy team will re-evaluate Bob's needs in a long-term care setting, in discussion with Bob's family and the multi-disciplinary team (MDT)

- nursing staff to provide the family with a list of care homes that specialise in dementia care and are near to them
- MDT to discuss Bob's progress with his family and explain the strategies that help him best

---

Box XVIII.i   A therapist's perspective

In dementia settings, some of the 'traditional' Occupational Therapy assessments can be inappropriate when trying to capture a person's remaining level of function, as we are dealing with people whose performance is strongly impaired. So, it is often the family members that we have the most conversations with. They are worried about their parent or their spouse, and we can get some very conflicting views about what should be happening. As a result, the occupational therapist and the care coordinator are responsible for pulling together all kinds of strands of information to ensure the situation is treated holistically and all bases are covered; and it would be really easy to lose the person's voice amongst all the generic work and the differing family opinions.

Formulation ensures that 'who the person is' – their identity – does not get swamped in the busyness of the generic work. And I think it helps with Capacity assessments when we have to be sure we are doing what the person would have wanted if they had the capacity to make the decision on their own – because it helps us to get to know the person as an occupational being.

Table XVIII.i Components of Bob's occupational identity

Roles/relationships	worked as shepherd and farm manager; lived with his wife, Alwynne, on a smallholding; close bond with sheepdog; coped with the long hours and unpredictable routines – washing hands in streams & troughs, and changing overalls indoors
Turning points (inc., changes to physical & social environments)	brought up on a farm; admitted to assessment unit with a chest infection, ear infection and cellulitis
Interests	enjoyed outdoor life, walking and reading non-fiction; attending village social events with wife; liked own company and keeping busy with jobs
Volition *(inc., appraisal of ability, expectation of success, values, choices, satisfaction & goals)*	private, stoic and independent; preferring to 'get by' without help and keep difficulties to self; quiet, reserved, placid; took great care to ensure welfare of animals; used to being own boss and supervising work of farmhands; initially unsettled and angry towards staff and frustrated by any interventions; inclined to participate in work-like activities; prefers to be in quiet places, e.g., courtyard

Table XVIII.ii Components of Bob's occupational competence

Routines	often takes his meals to eat on his own; was wakeful and agitated at night but now settled – going to bed at midnight, rising at 5 AM and napping occasionally; always doing something
Skills	appears not to recognise wife and children; keeps self to himself and does not relate to others spontaneously; responsive to therapeutic interaction; shows humour at times; physically strong with imposing stature; independently mobile despite unsteady gait due to swollen feet; becomes focused on tasks; difficulty hearing others
Performance	was sitting with his eyes closed; often gets up and walks away when family visit; looks at farming magazines and a photo of favourite sheepdog; eats well and can be prompted to participate in self-care activities; undresses and urinates in public areas at times and resists staff intervention, becoming physically and verbally aggressive; has inadvertently damaged objects or caused obstructions – taking cushion pads out of covers and trying to put covers back on, moving walking frames, and attempting to mend objects
Environmental contexts	wife admitted to hospital following a fall; residential home was unable to cope with his needs; large, supportive family but assessment unit is far from them and his home; OT support staff initiate interaction; staff attempt to maintain his dignity; ward environment is specifically designed for people with dementia and facilitates walking around the unit

References

Cooper J, Parkinson S, De les Heras de Pablo CG, Shute R, Melton J, Forsyth K (2018) *A User's Manual for the Model of Human Occupation Exploratory Level Outcome Ratings (MOHO-ExpLOR) Version 1.0*. Edinburgh: NHS Lothian and Queen Margaret University.

Kielhofner G, Mallinson T, Crawford C, Nowak M, Rigby M, Henry A, Walens D (2004) *Occupational Performance History Interview (OPHI-II) Version 2.1*. Chicago: University of Illinois.

XIX Occupational Therapy in a learning disability day service

– an example occupational formulation with measurable goals

Overview

Here is another occupational formulation which has been informed by the Model of Human Occupation Exploratory Level Outcome Ratings (MOHO-ExpLOR). In this case, Prakesh is less able to verbalise his feelings and intentions, and so his volition must be inferred from his actions and volitional behaviours. For instance, it is inferred that he has a close relationship with his grandmother and a good relationship with his carers because of his actions, and it is inferred that he is anxious about new activities and enjoys other activities because of his volitional behaviours. It takes time to gather and confirm this information and so the occupational therapist involves Prakesh in exploratory interventions, requiring a single step in a task, to gain a better understanding of his volition and his ability.

The occupational therapist has indicated which of the key issues are related to how Prakesh is behaving, and which concern his family's actions. The therapist then proceeds to set goals for Prakesh to achieve when the issues relate to his behaviour, and to negotiate a measurable goal with his family when their actions are the focus of the issue. Unusually, the timeframe for all three goals is the same – 6 months – suggesting that change is likely to be slow, and that Prakesh is unlikely to benefit from having varied timeframes, because he would be unable to comprehend something as abstract as a goal. In fact, all the interventions relating to the first two issues are to be completed by the occupational therapist, and yet she has still managed to write the goals in such a way that they focus on what Prakesh will achieve.

Notice how:
- the Volitional Questionnaire (de las Heras et al. 2007) is used to gather information and reveals how spontaneous Prakesh is in the following

  o *showing curiosity* – when puppets are used to initiate interaction
  o *Initiating actions* – when following verbal and visual prompts
  o *trying new things* – when he has gained confidence with people
  o *showing preferences* – when his 'Nani' is mentioned
  o *showing that an activity is special* - when motivated by food and drink

- the key occupational issues are linked to the people in question
- all the initial and the successive goals have been set for 6 months
- the interventions are largely to be completed by the occupational therapist, but Prakesh, his family, and his carers, remain the subjects of the goals

---

DOI: 10.4324/9781003046301-119

Introduction

Prakesh is a 25-year-old man with moderate to severe learning disabilities and autism, and who has a history of engaging in self-injurious behaviours. He was referred by Social Care services to Occupational Therapy to assess and treat his sensory needs

Occupational assessments completed:

- Model of Human Occupation Exploratory Level Outcome Ratings (Cooper et al. 2018)
- Volitional Questionnaire (de las Heras et al. 2007)
- Structured observations of graded task performance
- Informal interviews with family and carers during a home visit

Occupational identity

Prakesh lives with his mum and dad (aged 45 and 50 respectively), his 'Nani' (maternal grandmother, aged 75), an older brother, and a younger sister aged 10. He also has another sister with additional learning disability and physical needs who is currently living in residential care. His parents both work long hours in the family shop and Prakesh appears to have a strong attachment to his Nani. Although Prakesh's communication is almost entirely non-verbal and often unclear, his feelings may be inferred from his actions. For instance, he smiles and makes a happy-sounding scream when Nani is mentioned. He also seems to have a good relationship with his carers – pulling them into the occupational therapy sessions, readily allowing them to sit next to him, and willingly going out into the community with them.

He becomes anxious when new activities are introduced and may seek reassurance in the presence of trusted others, but may also scream and kick or attempt to engage in self-injurious behaviours – mostly banging his head and scratching or pinching his body – and will rock repeatedly. He is also reluctant to try different sensations and does not like showers or baths or having his hair cut. He habitually tucks his arms inside his clothing to avoid touch, but is strongly motivated to reach out for food and drink, and maintains an emotional connection to activities that he enjoys. Although he does not actively pursue any interests, he appears content when out walking and when visiting local parks and cafés, and his grandmother says he enjoys watching his siblings kicking a football in the garden. In therapy sessions, he laughs when puppets are used to initiate interaction.

Occupational competence

Prakesh's mum deals with the family finances and Prakesh spends much of his time in the company of his Nani, who takes most of the responsibility for helping Prakesh with self-care tasks such as preparing food for Prakesh and ensuring that Prakesh takes liquid medications, which are given to him in his food and drink. Prakesh does not assist with any household tasks and sleeps in a chair in the sitting room rather than going to bed. He has few belongings of his own, other than clothing, having broken things that he has been given in the past. Carers visit every weekday and take Prakesh out for walks. They have not attempted to kick a football with Prakesh, but confirm that his mobility is good and that he can walk for several miles at a time.

Prakesh will try new experiences with people he has gained confidence with, and responds well to intensive interaction techniques. For instance, he often clicks his teeth and when the occupational therapist replies by clicking her teeth, he appears to recognise that the communication is two-way. Over time, he has followed demonstrated actions and responded to visual aids and verbal prompts to complete one-step tasks. These involve taking his arms out of his clothing and opening a cookie jar, putting rubbish in a bin, or holding the juice carton when having a drink. He appears to remember where things are kept and what will happen next in a sequence of actions.

Key occupational issues

- Prakesh – communicating with others
- Prakesh – using hands to complete personal and domestic ADL tasks
- family and carers – extending opportunities for Prakesh

Summary statement

Prakesh is strongly attached to his Nani (grandmother), has a good relationship with carers, is motivated by food, and responds well to intensive interaction techniques.

He is gaining confidence with the occupational therapists, and he would benefit from building relationships with others. He habitually tucks his arms inside his clothing to avoid tactile sensations, but can be encouraged to use his hands to complete small ADL tasks. At the moment, his routine is limited to going for walks and it will be important to work with family and carers to extend future opportunities.

Initial goals and interventions

1a. Over the next 6 months, Prakesh will explore ways to communicate with others, with invitations and prompting from the occupational therapist (OT)

- OT to pursue intensive intervention techniques and playful use of puppets to initiate interaction
- OT to explore sensory techniques with Prakesh, including the use of the glider swing prior to activities, to modulate his sensory needs
- OT to liaise with the Speech and Language Therapist regarding the best communication strategies
- OT to create and trial a range of visual communication aids

2a. Over the 6 months, Prakesh will practise using his hands to complete tasks for Activities of Daily Living in therapy sessions with graded structure and activity analysis by the occupational therapist

- OT to introduce a range of tactile sensations, using food as a motivator
- OT to assess Prakesh's ability to complete a range of 1-step tasks relating to personal and domestic Activities of Daily Living

3a. Over the next 6 months, Prakesh's family and carers will identify ways to extend opportunities for Prakesh, with suggestions and guidance by the occupational therapist

- OT to get to know Prakesh's family's needs and discuss the possibility of introducing new objects for Prakesh to interact with at home

- OT to explore leisure interests with Prakesh and discuss opportunities to involve Prakesh with family and carers
- OT to review opportunities for Prakesh to interact with peers and assess his ability to tolerate interaction with new people

Successive goals and interventions

1b. Over the next 6 months, Prakesh will practise ways to communicate with others, with encouragement from and modelling by the occupational therapist

- OT to model agreed communication strategies with carers and family who attend therapy sessions

2b. Over the next 6 months, Prakesh will practise using his hands to complete ADL tasks outside of the therapy sessions, as demonstrated by the occupational therapist in negotiation with family and carers

- OT to assess Prakesh's ability to complete a range of two-step tasks relating to personal and domestic Activities of Daily Living
- OT to introduce water play with a proprioceptive-rich element and explore ways to make washing/bathing more comfortable for Prakesh
- carers to introduce increased opportunities for physical activity when taking Prakesh out

3b. Over the next 6 months, Prakesh's family and carers will plan ways to extend opportunities for Prakesh, with coaching by the occupational therapist

- Prakesh to be offered choices between two items in cafes, to carry items to the table and to help tidy away
- OT and family to discuss ways of making Prakesh's bedroom more inviting
- OT to talk to Prakesh's family's about their long-term expectations of living with Prakesh

Box XIX.i   A therapist's perspective

In my experience, learning disability colleagues often focus on problems such as: what the person requires help with and what additional needs they may have. Creating occupational formulations has helped me to promote a person's skills and interests, and the positives in their life. More than this, I find that it has encouraged me to explore areas that I might have otherwise overlooked; for example, by cultivating a person's interests when they have been unable to identify any, even though this was not the reason for referral and carers have not identified leisure as a cause of concern.

When I was first introduced to occupational formulation, it was tricky to organise the relevant information into the framework, especially when compiling information for someone who has numerous life complications. Focusing on the individual components of a formulation allowed me to organise the information as it emerged during the assessment process, and helped me to pick out the important bullet points before putting them into the formulation. Overall, I think completing case formulations assists me to focus on the core principles of OT, to build a truly holistic picture of the person, and to develop person-centred goals.

Table XIX.i Components of Prakesh's occupational identity

Roles/relationships	lives with mum (45) and dad (50), his 'Nani' (75), an older brother, and younger sister (10); has another sister with learning and physical needs in residential care; has good relationship with carers
Turning points (inc., changes to physical & social environments)	Nani (maternal grandmother) is aging
Interests	does not actively pursue interests but appears content when out walking, visiting local parks and cafés; grandmother says he enjoys watching siblings play with football; laughs when puppets are used to initiate interaction
Volition *(inc., appraisal of ability, expectation of success, values, choices, satisfaction & goals)*	appears to have a strong attachment to his Nani – smiles and makes a happy-sounding scream when she is mentioned; also seems to have good relationship with carers – pulling them into OT sessions, willingly sitting next to them and going out with them; becomes anxious when new activities are introduced - seeking reassurance from others; reluctant to try different sensations and does not like showers or baths or having his hair cut; habitually tucks his arms inside clothing to avoid touch; strongly motivated by food and drink and maintains an emotional connection to activities he enjoys

Table XIX.ii Components of Prakesh's occupational competence

Routines	parents both work long hours in the family shop; Prakesh spends much of his time in the company of his Nani; carers visit every weekday; sleeps in a chair in the sitting room rather than a bed
Skills	communication is almost entirely non-verbal and often unclear- feelings may be inferred from actions; often mishandles objects and breaks them but mobility is good – walking for several miles; responds well to intensive interaction techniques (e.g., clicking teeth); remembers where things are kept and what will happen next in a sequence of actions
Performance	may scream, kick or self-injure – banging head and scratching or pinching body – and will rock repeatedly when anxious; takes liquid medications in food and drink; does not assist with household tasks; will try new experiences with trusted others; has followed demonstrated actions, inc., visual aids and verbal prompts to complete one-step tasks – taking arms out of clothing, opening cookie jar, putting rubbish in bin, or holding juice carton
Environmental contexts	Prakesh's mum deals with family finances and, Nani helps Prakesh with self-care including feeding; Prakesh has few belongings of his own, (other than clothing); family have not attempted to play football with him; take him out for walks

References

Cooper J, Parkinson S, De les Heras de Pablo CG, Shute R, Melton J, Forsyth K (2018) *A User's Manual for the Model of Human Occupation Exploratory Level Outcome Ratings (MOHO-ExpLOR) version 1.0*. Edinburgh: NHS Lothian and Queen Margaret University.

de las Heras, CG. Geist, R. Kielhofner, G. Li Y (2007) *A user's guide to the Volitional Questionnaire (VQ) version 4.1*. Chicago: University of Illinois.

XX Occupational Therapy in a community learning disability service

– an example occupational formulation with measurable goals

Overview

Following this example of a formulation and goals, a sample progress report has been added (see Table XX.ii), so that you can see how the formulation and goals can both be used to inform subsequent reports.

The assessments on which the formulation was based would have contained a lot of detailed information, and would generally have been presented as a list of assessed items. Lists can be difficult to absorb, and assessment items tend to include specialist terms that may not be clearly understood by a non-specialist. A formulation, on the other hand, is able to take the findings of multiple assessments to create a story that has a beginning (the person's identity), a middle (the person's competence), and a conclusion (the presenting issues). More than this, it is packed with personal details that bring the story to life and make it memorable, and ensure that the formulation focuses on the person rather than the therapist's own analysis.

Assessments and formulations complement each other. One could be forgiven for thinking that some assessments are primarily for the therapist's benefit, as they help the therapist to gather information systematically in order to develop their analysis; whereas formulations benefit the person more because they give the person a voice and lead to person-centred goals. Yet, occupational formulations are based on the assessments, and both are important for ensuring that therapy makes a difference to the person. While the formulations may lead to person-centred goals and measures of goal attainment, standardised assessments can also be repeated and used as outcome measures. Together, they provide better feedback for the individual and better evidence regarding the effectiveness of Occupational Therapy.

Introduction

Wendy is a 46-year-old lady with a Learning Disability. Wendy was referred to Occupational Therapy via the community nursing team for an assessment of her support needs:

Formal occupational assessments completed:
- Occupational Self Assessment (OSA) (Baron et al. 2006)
- Assessment of Motor and Process Skills (AMPS) (Fisher and Jones 2014)
- Assessment of Communication and Interaction Skills (ACIS) (Forsyth et al. 1998)
- Model of Occupation Screening Tool (MOHOST) (Parkinson et al. 2006)

DOI: 10.4324/9781003046301-120

> **Notice how:**
> - the occupational therapist has made a thorough assessment of Wendy's needs before composing the occupational formulation, and has divided the assessments according to whether they are formal or informal
> - whereas the assessment summaries might report on Wendy's strengths and limitations in terms of her volition, habituation, skills, performance and participation, and her environmental context, the formulation integrates all the assessment information into a narrative, making it easier to comprehend
> - information from the formulation and the single observation MOHOST have been used to create an Occupational Therapy progress report, which includes Wendy's latest goals and a descriptive account of her achievements

Informal occupational assessments completed:
- Activities of Daily Living Assessment

Occupational identity

Wendy has lived all her life in a bungalow with her mum. They are happy living together and have a very good relationship. Wendy also talks with affection about her dad who had Alzheimer's, and who passed away a few years ago after moving into a care home. Her brother and half-sister live close by and she says that she gets on with her brother but that her relationship with her half-sister is 'up and down'. She sometimes feels that her half-sister criticises her, thinks she is 'stupid', and 'tells her what to do', which she does not like. Yet despite not always getting on with her half-sister, Wendy talks fondly of her family and appreciates the support that they offer.

Wendy's mum, Joyce, is 85 and has become very unwell in recent months, so Wendy is caring for her. She values this role as it makes her feel that she is helping, and she would not want anyone else to do it. Ideally, she would like to continue to live in the bungalow with her mum. She is afraid of any outside help from services because she does not want others to know that she is struggling, and she is worried her mum will be taken into care. Sometimes, she feels 'useless' because she wants to be able to do everything independently and feels upset when she cannot. For example, she has never done much cooking because this was always Joyce's role, and she would like to learn how to do this.

Wendy has volunteered at a Charity shop two days a week for approximately 30 years, and says that she enjoys this but that it can be stressful and feel overwhelming at times. In the past, she used to enjoy organised coach trips and holidays with her mum and she still enjoys going out to lunch with her mum.

Occupational competence

Wendy and her mum offer each other mutual support and they have managed well for many years. Until recently, Wendy supported her mum with physical tasks because her mum's mobility had deteriorated, while Joyce supported Wendy with verbal reminders to do the housework. However, as her mum has become more unwell, Wendy has become her full-time caregiver and now helps her with washing, dressing, and transferring on and off the toilet. Also, because Joyce always took full responsibility for cooking, Wendy is now learning to heat up ready-made meals. She is well-oriented to her kitchen, so can select and find appropriate equipment and utensils. She needs support to know when fresh produce is still alright to eat, and how to check food dates and cooking instructions.

Wendy has adequate skills to manage familiar day-to-day tasks including shopping and doing laundry. She has difficulty completing cleaning tasks to a sufficiently high standard and so her sister assists when necessary - often when Wendy is out of the house. Wendy also finds more complex things difficult to understand, such as her mum's medication, information from the GP, and money management. When her sister attempts to offer suggestions Wendy can interpret this as criticism, however, she will ask for her sister's help if she becomes confused by certain letters or phone calls. She knows that she could also call on her brother, although he has his own health problems and has infrequent contact.

Wendy is a very friendly, polite, and cheerful woman, with good communication skills. She presents as being very capable and she once completed some self-assessment forms to reflect this, which led to her benefits being removed as a consequence. She does not have any of her own friends or a support network, and has so far declined to join groups in her area. She has always socialised with her mum and her mums' friends, and as Joyce is becoming more unwell, their trips out are becoming more infrequent. Wendy has also reduced her hours to two mornings a week at the charity shop so she can be at home with her mum. She benefits from a high level of support and reassurance to complete delegated tasks at the shop, such as sorting through donated items, wiping down shelves, and hanging up clothes.

Key occupational issues

- developing meal preparation skills
- managing household tasks
- building a social life and support network
- anticipating future needs

Summary statement

Wendy is a friendly, polite, and cheerful woman who volunteers at a charity shop and is keen to help her mum, Joyce. She is currently helping Joyce with all aspects of her personal care.

Joyce always used to do the cooking and Wendy is beginning to develop skills for meal preparation. She also manages most household tasks with occasional help from her sister. She used to enjoy coach trips with Joyce and would benefit from greater social support. Meanwhile, Wendy wants to stay living with her mum as long as possible, but her future needs will need further assessment.

Initial goals

1a over the next 6 weeks, Wendy will practise meal preparation skills in her own home, with instruction and supervision from the Occupational Therapy assistant

2a within the next 4 weeks, Wendy will re-evaluate the assistance she needs with household tasks, with feedback and suggestions from the occupational therapist

3a over the next 8 weeks, Wendy will explore a range of opportunities for building a social life and social network, with direction and advice from the occupational therapist

4a over the next 3 months, Wendy will negotiate her future needs with continued support from her sister and guidance from the occupational therapist

---

Box XX.i   A therapist's perspective

Prior to training in occupational formulation and measurable goals by Sue Parkinson, I had not completed a formulation of any kind, nor was it a familiar tool, despite the fact that I had experience of using MOHO in my work.

As I have a tendency to 'waffle', I found it useful to separate out the information I had gathered regarding the client into the various components before drafting a formulation. It also helped to keep the information succinct and relevant to what was required. It ensured that the information I was including remained occupation-focused rather than including details that may sit under a different profession's analysis.

Using the formulation process encourages the individuals' strengths and positives to be central to the analysis. Although difficulties and challenges to occupational performance are identified, after using this process I found that my interpretation of a client identified more positives in her abilities and her environment.

It was a concern that using the formulation process might be a more time-consuming approach and would increase workload. However, once familiar with the layout, it assisted in keeping paperwork focused and relevant. It has helped to streamline the Occupational Therapy process within the team, structure our reports and assessments, and encouraged us to use standardised approaches to assessment.

It is hoped that in the future this approach is used more consistently across the service, and will ensure a consistent approach to working with all clients.

Table XX.i Components of Wendy's occupational identity

Roles/relationships	has lived all her life in a bungalow with her mum; brother and half-sister live close by; currently caring for mum; has volunteered at a charity shop for about 30 years
Turning points (inc., changes to physical & social environments)	dad passed away a few years ago; mum is 85 and has become very unwell, and Wendy is struggling with caring role and independent living tasks – mum used to do all the cooking
Interests	enjoys volunteer role; used to enjoy organised coach trips and holidays with mum, and still enjoys going to out to lunch with mum
Volition *(inc., appraisal of ability, expectation of success, values, choices, satisfaction & goals)*	happy living with Mum and has very good relationship; talks fondly of Dad; gets on with brother – less so with half-sister who she describes being critical; appreciates all family support and values role as carer but worried her mum will go into care; sometimes feels useless – wants to do everything - feels upset when she cannot; would like to learn how to cook

Table XX.ii Components of Wendy's occupational competence

Routines	trips out with mum are becoming more infrequent; has reduced volunteer role to two mornings a week, to be at home with mum
Skills	well orientated to kitchen; selects and finds equipment and utensils; has adequate skills to manage day-to-day familiar tasks; finds complex things difficult to understand; may interpret suggestions as criticism; generally, is very friendly, polite and cheerful with good communication skills
Performance	managed well for many years with mum's help; supported mum with physical tasks as mum's mobility deteriorated; now assists mum with washing, dressing, and transferring on and off the toilet; learning to heat up ready-made meals; needs support to check food dates and cooking instructions; manages shopping and laundry; struggles with mum's medication, information from the GP, and money management; will ask sister to help with letters and phone calls; once had benefits removed because she presents as capable and filled in claim form to reflect this; sorts through donated items, wipes down shelves, and hangs up clothes at charity shop
Environmental contexts	mum supported with verbal reminders to do housework; sister attempts to offer suggestions; brother has health problems and has infrequent contact; no friends or a support network, and has declined groups in her area; benefits from high level of support and reassurance at the charity shop

Table XX.iii Progress Report

Occupational Therapy Progress Report

Full name: *Wendy* Date of birth:
Address:

Postcode:
ID code: Preferred name:
Occupational Therapist's name: Date: [4 months after initial goals agreed]
Signature: Base:

Introduction

Wendy is a 46 year old lady with a Learning Disability. Wendy was referred to Occupational Therapy via the community nursing team for an assessment of her support needs:

Formal Assessments: Occupational Self Assessment (OSA) (Baron et al. 2006); Assessment of Motor and Process Skills (AMPS) (Fisher and Jones 2014); Assessment of Communication and Interaction Skills (ACIS) (Forsyth et al. 1998); Model of Occupation Screening Tool (MOHOST) (Parkinson et al. 2006)

Informal Assessments: Activities of Daily Living Assessment

Summary of case formulation dated ___ / ___ / ___

Wendy is a friendly, polite and cheerful woman who volunteers at a charity shop and is keen to help her mum, Joyce. She is currently helping Joyce with all aspects of her personal care. Joyce always used to do the cooking and Wendy is beginning to develop skills for meal preparation. She also manages most household tasks with occasional help from her sister. She used to enjoy coach trips with Joyce and would benefit from greater social support. In addition, her future needs will need further assessment as Wendy wants to stay living with her mum as long as possible.

Key occupational issues

1 developing meal preparation skills
2 managing household tasks
3 building a social life and support network
4 anticipating future needs

Current goals

1b Over the next 3 months, Wendy will practise meal preparation skills in her own home with verbal prompts from the Occupational Therapy assistant
2b Over the next 3 months, Wendy will plan how to manage and practise agreed household tasks with advice from the occupational therapist
3b Over the next 2 months, Wendy will identify the most suitable opportunities for building a social life and social network, with encouragement from the occupational therapist
4b Over the 4 months, Wendy will explore options for meeting her future needs in negotiation with her sister and with guidance from the occupational therapist

Intervention summary

• Meal preparation practice, including chopping, boiling, steaming, microwaving and storing food
• Sourcing simpler microwave
• Creation of visual recipe cards and notices with instructions for household tasks
• Agreeing weekly timetable for shopping, laundry and cleaning, and practising these
• Liaison with charity shop regarding volunteer role

- Visiting local groups that offer social outings and lunch clubs
- Working with Wendy's sister to find best ways to offer feedback to Wendy
- Liaison with Wendy's sister regarding her mother's changing health needs

Achievements to date   Date ___ / ___ / ___
- expressing greater confidence in abilities
- more willing to accept help and accept feedback
- beginning to trust occupational therapist and voice preferences
- showing greater care in task completion and following visual instructions well
- more able to handle equipment efficiently and effectively
- able to make simple meals using the microwave, load a washing machine and complete dusting and vacuuming following a weekly schedule
- has shown interest in an outings group and a lunch club, viewing these as future options, rather than current possibilities
- has agreed tasks that are within her abilities and tasks that she can delegate to her sister

Outcome measure:	Baseline ratings	Outcome ratings
Single observation MOHOST	**Date:**	**Date:**
assessing meal preparation skills		
Motivation for occupation	**9/16**	**12/16**
Pattern of occupation	**9/16**	**11/16**
Communication & Interaction	**11/16**	**13/16**
Process skills	**8/16**	**12/16**
Motor skills	**13/16**	**14/16**
Environment	**13/16**	**14/16**

Goal Attainment																				
Goal number	\multicolumn 1					2					3					4				
	a	b	c	d	e	a	b	c	d	e	a	b	c	d	e	a	b	c	d	e
Much more than expected																				
More than expected	✓																			
As expected						✓										✓				
Less than expected											✓									
Much less than expected																				

To show that this form has been worked through with service user
Signature of service user:

References

Baron K, Kielhofner G, Iyenger A, Goldhammer V, Wolenski J (2006) *A User's Manual for the Occupational Self Assessment (OSA) Version 2.2*. Chicago: University of Illinois.

Fisher AG, Jones KB (2014) *Assessment of motor and process skills. Vol 2: User manual* (8th ed.) Fort Collins, CO: Three Stars Press.

Forsyth K, Salamy M, Simon S, Kielhofner G (1998) *The Assessment of Communication and Interaction Skills (ACIS) Version 4.0*. Chicago: University of Illinois.

Parkinson S, Forsyth K, Kielhofner G (2006) *The Model of Human Occupation Screening Tool (MOHOST) Version 2.0*. Chicago: University of Illinois.

Outline of the range of occupational issues in example occupational formulations

Example 1 – Emma
Paediatric Service
- taking part in organised physical activities
- working at a desk
- making the most of break times
- calming down when upset

Example 2 – Lucy
Children's Mental Health Service
- doing things she likes
- looking after herself
- having a family life
- continuing with her education

Example 3 – Mick
Adolescent Mental Health Service
- coping with bus journeys
- maintaining social conversation
- completing your college course
- finding a social outlet for your interests

Example 4 – Jessica
Perinatal Mental Health Service
- establishing self as a confident mother
- re-establishing self-care
- regaining physical fitness
- rediscovering motivation for interests

Example 5 – Sam
Acute Mental Health Service
- spending time outdoors
- revising mother/son role
- considering future work options
- finding a sense of community

Example 6 – Rebecca
Primary Care Service
- developing new interests
- finding a meaningful primary role
- having quality time with family
- forming valued social relationships

Example 7 – Linda
Community Mental Health Service
- preparing food in her kitchen
- uncovering and displaying antique sewing machines
- finding a social outlet for craft interests

Example 8 – Marcia
Mental Health Rehabilitation Service
- involvement in garden-based activities
- independence in everyday tasks
- developing respectful relationships
- pain management

Example 9 – Gary
Secure Mental health Service
- enhancing role within the family
- going to college to study music
- developing skills to manage independent living

Example 10 – Arran
Prison Service
- maximising family involvement
- obtaining future work
- practising everyday activities
- finding energy for active leisure interests

Example 11 – Brian
Service for Homeless People
- having own place to live
- maintaining mental health and self-care
- using interests to gain work
- establishing a support network

Example 12 – Banita
Traumatic Stress Service
- getting to know people
- expressing true self
- developing skills

Example 13 – Saaid
Independent Vocational Service
- mobility at work
- office dynamics
- work/life balance

Example 14 – Courtney
Acute Physical Service
- getting in and out of bed
- washing and dressing lower body
- re-establishing role as mum

Example 15 – Richard
Community Reablement Service
- contributing to the home and family
- regaining physical fitness to play golf
- maintaining a loving relationship as a husband

Example 16 – Frances
Adult Social Care Service
- adapting downstairs accommodation
- enabling wheelchair access to the front door
- advising about funding for future needs

Example 17 – Mr J
Intermediate Care Services
- returning to going out on mobility scooter
- returning to previous interests and hobbies
- adapting home environment
- managing personal care

Example 18 – Bob
Dementia Assessment Service
- establishing clear communication
- maintaining Bob's dignity
- involving Bob in work-like activities
- identifying a long-term care setting

Example 19 – Prakesh
Learning Disability Day Service
- communicating with others
- using hands to complete personal and domestic ADL tasks
- extending opportunities for Prakesh

Example 20 – Wendy
Community Learning Disability Service
- developing meal preparation skills
- managing household tasks
- building a social life and support network
- anticipating future needs

Index

Printed in the United States
by Baker & Taylor Publisher Services